—How can I be sure I have cystitis?
—Why do I get cystitis so often?
—How will cystitis affect my sex life?
—Is my diaphragm causing my cystitis?
—Can a change in diet prevent an attack?
—Does cranberry juice really help?
—How can I find the right doctor?
—What medical tests will I have to take?
—Which drugs work best?

Dr. Kathryn Schrotenboer Cox expertly and sensitively answers these and many more questions about the physical aspects of cystitis, its psychological impact, how you can get the help you need today—and prevent recurrences tomorrow.

THE WOMAN DOCTOR'S GUIDE TO OVERCOMING CYSTITIS

KATHRYN SCHROTENBOER COX, M.D., is an attending obstetrician and gynecologist at the New York Hospital/ Cornell Medical Center in New York City. She is editor of *Family Circle* magazine's popular column "Ask the Doctor," the author of *Dr. Kathryn Schrotenboer's Guide to Pregnancy Over 35*, and co-author of *Freedom From Menstrual Cramps*.

SUE BERKMAN is a pr[...]
have appeared in *Esquir*[...]
Mademoiselle.

D0711455

THE WOMAN DOCTOR'S GUIDE TO OVERCOMING CYSTITIS

Kathryn Schrotenboer Cox, M.D.
with Sue Berkman

A Smith and Kraus, Inc. Book

Illustrations by Logan Goodman

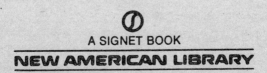

A SIGNET BOOK

NEW AMERICAN LIBRARY

Note to the Reader
The ideas, procedures, and suggestions contained in this book are not
intended as a substitute for consulting with your physician. All matters
regarding your health require medical supervision.

NAL BOOKS ARE AVAILABLE AT QUANTITY DISCOUNTS WHEN USED TO
PROMOTE PRODUCTS OR SERVICES. FOR INFORMATION PLEASE WRITE TO
PREMIUM MARKETING DIVISION, NEW AMERICAN LIBRARY, 1633
BROADWAY, NEW YORK, NEW YORK 10019.

 SIGNET TRADEMARK REG. U.S. PAT. OFF. AND FOREIGN COUNTRIES
REGISTERED TRADEMARK—MARCA REGISTRADA
HECHO EN DRESDEN, TN, U.S.A.

SIGNET, SIGNET CLASSIC, MENTOR, ONYX, PLUME,
MERIDIAN and NAL BOOKS are published by NAL PENGUIN
INC., 1633 Broadway, New York, New York 10019

First Signet Printing, June, 1989

1 2 3 4 5 6 7 8 9

PRINTED IN THE UNITED STATES OF AMERICA

*To my patients
and the millions
of cystitis sufferers*

ACKNOWLEDGMENTS

There are many people without whom this book might not have been written. For their help, we thank:

Lynne M. Perkins, R.D., M.S., M.A., for her valuable professional advice on the role of diet;

Dagmar O'Connor, Director of the Sexual Therapy Program at St. Luke's–Roosevelt Hospital Center, for helping to put the sex factor into focus;

Ann LaForge, for hours of exacting editing work;

Patricia and John Ford, for many drafts on many diskettes;

June Rosenberg, for retrieving data that would have taken months to find;

Terry Steinberg Elliot, for handling my many office affairs professionally and patiently when deadlines began to press;

The Interstitial Cystitis Association, for a wealth of straightforward information on a little-known disease;

Norwich–Eaton Pharmaceuticals, Roerig Pfizer, Riker Laboratories, Roche Laboratories, Ames Division of Miles Laboratories, Parke–Davis, Beecham Laboratories, National Women's Health Network, United States Department of Health, Education, and Welfare, Public Health Service, for supplying scientific studies, statistical information, and helpful suggestions;

Our family and friends, who always understood that the book came first.

Contents

Introduction

Several years ago I set as a personal goal to do all that I could to foster a physician/patient relationship that included openness and a sharing of information. I believe that women have always had the capacity to take responsibility for their own health care if only given the facts. The common thread and motivating factor in all of my publications to date, *Freedom From Menstrual Cramps*, *Pregnancy Over 35*, my contribution to *Everywoman's Health Guide*, as well as my "Ask the Doctor" column in *Family Circle* magazine, has been to help women to better understand how our bodies work. This book may not be glamorous in its subject material but it seeks to address a basic health concern that touches many of us as modern active women. There are many women with cystitis who may be suffering unnecessarily. I hope that this book will give them the information they need to work with their physicians to successfully overcome cystitis.

Kathryn Schrotenboer Cox, M.D.

PART I

UNDERSTANDING CYSTITIS

From Victim to Victor

Do you feel a sense of overwhelming frustration, a sense of helplessness about your recurring cystitis attacks?

Do you fear that sex will bring on a cystitis attack and, therefore, avoid it?

Is your discomfort making you irritable and nagging toward your family and friends?

Do you feel like you are being punished for something and don't know why?

Do you miss too many days of work?

Do you sometimes spend an entire sleepless night going from bed to bathroom and back again?

Do you refuse invitations for social engagements because you are having another attack?

If you answered "yes" to even one of the preceding questions, you may be a candidate for the cystitis prevention program. It offers a way out, maybe forever, from the limitations, burdens, fears, and doubts that cystitis has placed on your life.

What do you have to gain? Freedom from the physically devastating and emotionally debilitating disorder that robs you of perfect health and peace of mind.

ARE YOU READY?

The choice is yours. Are you ready to take a positive approach to prevention of cystitis? Your personalized program—the only one that will work perfectly for you—must start with three basic steps.

- First, gain all of the knowledge you can about the cause of your problem. In the first part of this book, you will learn every known fact about cystitis. You will learn about your genitourinary system, the organisms that cause the cystitis infection, the factors that increase the likelihood of infection setting in, the common symptoms, and how cystitis is diagnosed. You'll also learn what else besides cystitis could cause specific symptoms.
- Second, know the benefits of prevention. This means more than simply being aware that your actions will help you avoid the wretched symptoms of cystitis. It also means understanding the likelihood of cystitis developing into something far worse. You will learn the complications of cystitis in the first part of the book.
- Third, expect to customize the basic pattern laid out in this book. In many cases, you will read how other women have adapted the pattern to fit their own lifestyles and needs. Maybe some of their revisions meet your own requirements, maybe not. The important thing to remember is that there is no cookie-cutter approach to solving your cystitis problem. You are unique, and so is your condition.

A COMMON PROBLEM

In *Dorland's Medical Dictionary*, the "Webster's Unabridged" of the medical profession, cystitis (sis-ti'-tis) is given a four-word definition: "inflammation of the bladder." The type of cystitis we'll be discussing in these pages, for the most part, is *bacterial cystitis*, which is basically a bladder inflammation caused by a bacterial infection.

The entry for cystitis in Dorland's details many forms that the condition can take. For example, there is *cystitis cystica*, which is marked by the presence of translucent cysts in the bladder, and *interstitial cystitis*, an increasingly common condition whose cause is still unknown and that often progresses to ulceration and destruction of the bladder wall. There are also *diphtheritic cystitis*, *glandularis cystitis*, and *papiliomatosa*—all of which would make a simple bacterial infection pale by comparison.

Indeed, bacterial cystitis seems straightforward and unremarkable when compared with many of the disorders to which the entire urinary tract is prey. Consider urethritis, kidney stones, glomerulonephritis, nephrosis—all very serious diseases. It's little wonder that bacterial cystitis has been subjected to a short attention span from both gynecologists and urologists.

A LONG HISTORY

Infections of the urinary tract are no newcomers to the list of human sufferings. Even early civilizations were familiar with such afflictions; the healers of the time looked to urine for signs of disease. The word *cystitis* comes from the Greek *kystis*, meaning bladder, and *-itis*, which means inflammation. The ancients believed that this "flaming up" of the bladder was a punishment for evil, inflicted by the gods on any mortal with whom they were displeased.

Although we may no longer believe that cystitis is meted out from on high, it can seem like a form of punishment, particularly for a woman who is uninformed about the physiological aspects of the disease.

Stephanie R. is typical. A highly successful real estate consultant, 28 and single, she is clearly intelligent; yet she told me that her first attack of cystitis happened while she was in her early teens, about the time that she started to experience her own changing sexuality. "I honestly believed I was being punished for my sinful thoughts," she said.

Unfortunately, some people still seem to believe that cystitis is a woman's "lot in life."

Janet F., a 30-year-old potter, grew up in a family where the grandmother, mother and aunts all suffered from recurrent bouts of cystitis. "We all lived in the same small town, and it was impossible to go into any relative's house without hearing about someone doing something for a cystitis attack. I simply assumed that sooner or later I would have my first bout. Sure enough, at the age of 17, it happened. By that time, there were good drugs to cure the infection fast, so I didn't have to go through weeks of agony like the other women in my family had. But still, it would have been wonderful to know that I didn't have to suffer at all."

Cystitis can be an annoyance, a bother, a frustration, an irritation, and even a painful experience. Two things it is not, however, are punishment and an inevitable curse. Yet, time and again, I meet women who see it that way and, as a result, become victimized by the disease. In most instances, their attitudes are not a result of any conscious decisions. But their casual conversation carries the dispiriting story. "I had to give up my vacation," "I had to change my plans," and "I had to suffer through the trip," are statements that speak volumes.

Going from victim to victor may seem impossible to you if you have "given up," or "suffered through" for years. I can't recall a single woman who imagined that she could overcome the infection once and for all. But thousands have, and thousands more will. And so will you.

MISTAKEN IDEAS

In the spring of 1986, Merck Sharp & Dohme, a major pharmaceutical company, asked Gallup Organization pollsters to conduct a survey on women's awareness of urinary tract infections. The Gallup Organization interviewed 1,033 women by telephone and the questions yielded some surprising answers. I'd like to summarize the key findings here:

- *Almost half of all adult women have had an infection.* Almost half (43 percent) of the women reported having had a urinary tract infection at some time. One in 10 (9 percent) had an infection in the year prior to the survey. Another one in eight (12 percent) said their most recent occurrence was within the prior two to three years. Among those who had an infection during the previous year, most (82 percent) reported that they had experienced the problem once or twice within the year.
- *Most women do not know what causes urinary tract infections.* Approximately two-thirds (63 percent) of the women could not name a cause of urinary tract infections. Even among women who had had infection, nearly half (47 percent) could not name a cause. Ignorance among women who had never had an infection is even greater: Three out of four (74 percent) were unaware f the cause.
- *Many women are not aware of the symptoms of urinary tract infection.* When asked to name the symptoms of urinary tract infection, 37 percent could not name any. Women most likely to mention at least one symptom were those who had had an infection within the year past. The most frequently mentioned symptom was burning and pain during urination (51 percent). Next often mentioned was a need to urinate often.
- *Many women do not have a clear idea of how urinary*

tract infections are treated. One in three women (33 percent) could not name a treatment for urinary tract infections. Less than half reported that urinary tract infections are treated with antibiotics (41 percent). Others refer to medications in general. Less frequently mentioned are drinking large quantities of fluids (11 percent) or acidic juices such as cranberry or orange juice (4 percent). Women who have had the problem are more likely than those who have not had it to name at least one method of treatment.

• *Some women experience side effects from medication.* One in 10 (10 percent) women treated for a urinary tract infection reported experiencing side effects or adverse reactions from the medication. Among those who reported side effects, the most common problems appear to be nausea (25 percent) or rash (24 percent).

One of the most surprising results of the survey had to do with women's awareness of the prevalence of urinary tract infection. The women who were interviewed were read a list of four health problems—urinary tract infection, lung cancer, ovarian cysts, emphysema—and asked to indicate which of the four they believed women suffered most. Forty-seven percent correctly chose urinary tract infection. Incorrectly, 16 percent chose lung cancer, 12 percent chose ovarian cysts, 3 percent chose emphysema, and 1 percent chose breast cancer, which was the most frequently mentioned "other" response. In short, although nearly half of the women were aware that urinary tract infection was a leading health problem in women, the other half were *not* aware. Obviously, there is much to be done in terms of enlightening women as to how common urinary tract infection is.

There is much you can learn about the disease, why you get it, and what can be done about it.

I invite you to join me in the next chapter to start the task together.

CHAPTER 2

What You Can't See Can Hurt You

When I started out in the field of obstetrics and gynecology more than 10 years ago, the women's movement was in full flower. Women were being encouraged to know their own bodies, to take control of their own health, to participate in their own well-being.

Considering the progress that has been made, it always amazes me when women express so many uncertainties about the physical characteristics and the various systems that make them unique. Many women are uninformed about the most basic anatomical facts. There's confusion about where the kidneys are located, where the bladder lies, and what each of these organs does. Few women know how the organs function in *good* health, let alone when something goes wrong.

All this is not to say, however, that women aren't eager to learn. Over and over my patients tell me that gaining a clear picture of what is going on in their bodies makes them feel in control. Knowledge is the key to control. Knowing all about what is healthy and what is not is an important aspect of starting to reverse illness.

When Myrna B. began learning the simple physiological facts about her body, she was both excited and embarrassed. A woman of 41, Myrna had a teenage daughter, Joy, who seemed—to her mother at least—to be amazingly worldly. "How will I ever tell my daughter that I have been so much in the dark all these years?" Myrna asked one day.

As it turned out, Joy was in the dark too, and feeling the confusions of a young woman who is becoming aware of her own sexuality and her own body. Together Myrna and Joy made good use of the notes that Myrna had taken during our discussions together.

I hope that you will learn a great deal in the following pages, and that you will want to share some of the knowledge with others—your daughter, mother, best friend, or perhaps most important of all, your husband or lover.

A FOOLPROOF PROCESS

It's hard to imagine any body process more foolproof than that of urination. You drink a glass of milk or a cup of coffee, eat a piece of fruit, and before you know it, you have the urge to empty out all of the fluid that has collected in your body. The amazing thing is that most of the time the process *is* foolproof, you never have to think about it, you just respond when, as the expression goes, "nature calls." Considering the intricacies of the genitourinary system, it's surprising that something doesn't go wrong more often as fluid is maneuvered around and out of the body.

Let me take a minute to remind you that the external parts of the genitourinary system are part of the female genitals. They are not "private parts," "down there," "you know where," or any other euphemism. Nor is the product that passes out of your body when the genitourinary system works "number 1." It is urine. There is nothing wrong in calling bodily parts and processes by their rightful names.

Urination is only one of the many functions of the genitourinary system. It is necessary to put that particular function into context with the many other functions of the system. Only then can we speak of appearance, function, and process.

What follows is a simplified but thorough discussion of the female genitourinary system. To understand fully the terms and concepts, refer to the illustration on page 12, and try to locate the various elements in the system within your own body.

THE GENITOURINARY SYSTEM

The Kidneys

The genitourinary system begins with a pair of *kidneys*, which are situated on the back wall of the abdomen. There is one kidney on either side of the spine at about the level of the lowest rib (although the right kidney lies a little lower than the left). In an adult, each bean-shaped kidney is about 4 inches long, 2 ½ inches wide, and 1 ½ inches thick, and weighs about 5 ounces.

As part of its journey around the body, blood enters the kidneys through the renal arteries.

The kidneys are chemical processing works. There, waste matter in the blood is filtered out.

In the course of 24 hours, our kidneys filter a total of 180 quarts of fluid—and everything dissolved in it—out of the blood. With the exception of 1 to 1 ½ quarts of water (the normal amount of urine excreted in a day) all this fluid is reabsorbed, together with valuable substances such as sodium, potassium, and glucose. Only the waste products are left for excretion from the body, along with any salts that are in excess of what the body knows that it needs.

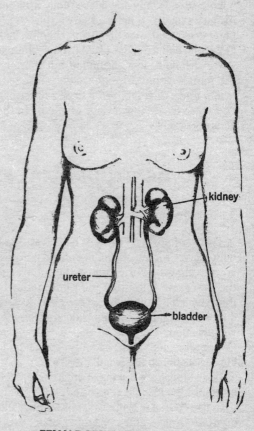

FEMALE GENITOURINARY SYSTEM

Once collected in the kidneys, urine is piped away through a long, hollow tube called a *ureter*. There is one ureter for each kidney. Each ureter is about the size of a strand of spaghetti. Through the ureters, the wastes reach a reservoir called the *bladder* (see illustration below).

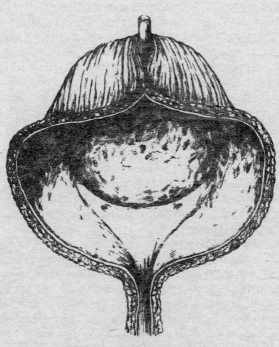

CROSS SECTION OF BLADDER

The Bladder

The bladder, probably because of its mundane chores, has never been considered a very glamorous organ. Indeed, it looks like a bag; when it is empty, it is flat; when it is full, it is rounded and projects upward. An adult bladder holds approximately 1.2 pints of urine—although the desire to urinate is often felt when the bladder is about half full.

The wall of the bladder is quite complex and highly sensitive. It is comprised of four layers: the outer or serous layer, the muscular layer, a submucosal layer that acts as connective tissue between adjoining layers, and the innermost mucosal layer. The bladder wall also has an efficient blood supply and lymphatic system, and is adequately supplied with nerves.

The Sphincters and Urethra

Fortunately for our state of ease and social convenience, the mechanical functions of the bladder are generally monitored, programmed, and operated with elegant efficiency. Indeed, to know something of these workings should command our respect.

At the bottom or neck of the bladder there is a collection of circular muscle fibers called the *internal sphincter*. An inch or so lower is the *external sphincter*. When the sphincters are contracted, urine cannot leak out of the bladder.

When urination occurs, the sphincters relax and the urine passes from the bladder to the *urethra* (see illustrations page 15). This is a muscular tube that measures about 1 ½ inches in length and is very straight in a woman. In a man, the urethra usually measures 8 inches in length, and is curved. Bearing that difference in mind will help you understand why women are so much more often the victims of bladder infections. The urethra leads to the exterior of the body. The process of urination is sometimes called voiding, or *micturition*.

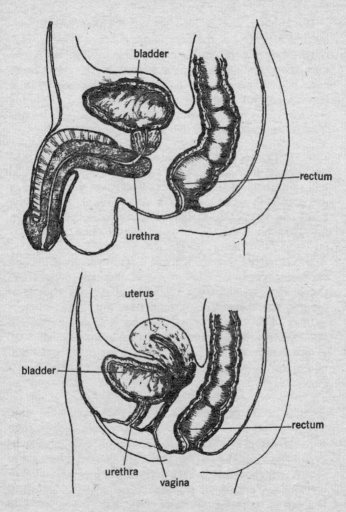

MALE AND FEMALE URETHRAS

The kidneys, ureters, bladder, and urethra are all primarily under control of the autonomic nervous system. This means that, like the cardiovascular system, respiratory system, and digestive system, the genitourinary system functions without our having to devote much thought to it, at least when it is functioning normally.

Voluntary Control

As any mother knows, there is no voluntary control of these bladder and urethral reflexes in infants. But ordinarily, a child will acquire an increasing ability to restrain the passage of urine, initially by day, and later also by night. The healthy adult who has acquired this voluntary control of the external sphincter is able to retain urine, even when the distended bladder is causing discomfort.

A further refinement of these elegant mechanisms is a reflex response to the effort to impose voluntary control when the opportunity to urinate is not available. This reflex temporarily suppresses the contractions of the bladder musculature and the urge to urinate decreases. This may happen several times before the urge becomes uncontrollable. All of this occurs without your giving it a momentary thought as you wait for the ideal opportunity to urinate.

A HOSTILE INVADER

In at least 85 percent of the women who have it, bacterial cystitis is caused by an organism called *Escherichia coli*, or *E. coli*, which normally lives in the lower intestine without causing any problems (see illustration page 17). In fact, it is essential to the normal functioning of the lower bowel. In smaller numbers *E. coli* is also present on the skin surrounding the vaginal area and in the vagina.

When *E. coli* manages to get into the bladder, which is

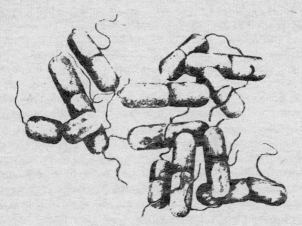

E. COLI

not difficult considering the short length of the urethra and the close proximity of the urethral opening to the vagina and the anus, it begins to act like an hostile invader. This causes the immune system to go into action, fighting the infection in much the same way it fights any other infection: White blood cells are deployed to search and destroy the marauding microorganisms.

Sometimes the battle is over quickly. Sometimes it becomes a long, drawn-out affair that causes fever and other related symptoms. Sometimes it is won only when the immune system is bolstered by reinforcements—drugs that are specifically developed to overcome the bacteria.

Normally, the whole urinary system is geared to rid itself of bacteria. When colonies of bacteria are deliberately inoculated into the bladders of experimental animals, all traces of them are frequently gone within 24 hours. And so it is with humans. Our urine, in a disease-free state, is sterile, free from bacteria and other contaminating organisms; the built-in safeguard that maintains this state of sterility in urination.

Unfortunately, bacteria seem to linger longer in female bladders than in males'. One reason is the pressure on a woman's bladder that occurs during sexual intercourse. This may impede the usual signals of the need to urinate.

A woman who wears a diaphragm may experience a similar reaction if the diaphragm presses firmly against the neck of her bladder.

Some women seem to be born with an exceptionally hospitable surface along the genitourinary tract. Researchers have begun to suspect that cystitis-prone women have cells lining their bladders that are more likely to allow bacteria to adhere than the bladders of women who are not prone to cystitis. At the same time, bacteria such as *E. coli* are found to have special structures called *pili*—something like sticky fingers—which search out areas that they can readily latch onto. Much research remains to be done in these new developments.

Another baffling aspect of bacterial cystitis is why normal urination does not eliminate all bacteria. The bladder is lined by *glycosaminoglycan* (GAG), which is highly efficient at reducing both bacterial adherence to the underlying mucosa and infection. Research points to the possibility that some women have a reduced quantity of GAG and, thus, are vulnerable to recurrent cystitis. Research in this area offers hope for a new type of antibacterial agent—one that works by augmenting the natural defense.

In the meantime, the primary reason for urine retention in the bladder is habit, not heredity or anatomy. (More on this in the next chapter.)

The Telltale Signs

When bacteria do gain a foothold in the bladder and cause cystitis, certain typical symptoms will herald the onset of the infection. Not every woman will experience all of these symptoms, nor will the symptoms occur to the same degree or intensity in every woman.

- Many women complain of a constant desire to urinate, even within seconds or minutes after having done so.
- Another complaint is a feeling of trying to force the urine out of the urethra.
- Women will also note a feeling of incomplete emptying of the bladder.
- Another common symptom is of considerable pain or burning upon urination. The pain, however, is not felt outside the urethral opening, but rather inside the urethra.
- With a majority of women, there is the need to urinate several times during the night. For this reason, some women think that their symptoms grow worse at night; quite likely it is because the symptoms interrupt sleep.
- Finally, there is a feeling of having a poor urinary stream —"Nothing but a little trickle," said one of my patients.

There are some other signs of cystitis: In some cases the appearance of the urine often changes as a result of infection. This may be the only notable abnormality in women who have the infection without the traditional symptoms. It is quite common for the urine to become cloudy, even milky, in appearance. Less often, the urine may appear reddish because of the presence of blood. (But both cloudy and bloody urine may stem from other causes as well.)

Fever, often associated with a chilly sensation, may accompany any or all of the other symptoms of cystitis. Fever is an important clue that the disease is actually an infection; often it is the ony sign of cystitis. Some women may experience nausea and vomiting along with the fever; this may, however, be in response to the fever rather than a primary symptom of the infection.

As intense as some of these sensations are, it is often difficult to describe them. And a precise description is just what a doctor needs in order to make a diagnosis. Pain, urgency, frequency, and so on may strongly suggest that there is a full-blown case of cystitis going on. Then again, the cause of the suffering may be something else entirely. For instance, pain during urination may be felt inside the urinary tract, which is a sign of bacterial cystitis, or it may be felt at the outside of the urinary tract, at the labia, or lips, which might indicate herpes or simply an irritation to the skin at that spot.

Learn to listen to your body, note the symptoms carefully, and write them down so that when you arrive for your appointment, ready for treatment, you and your doctor will both be sure that the treatment program is the best possible one for you.

COMMON PATTERNS

Sometimes the cystitis attacks fit into a certain pattern.

Isolated Episodes

An isolated episode of cystitis that clears spontaneously or readily responds to treatment is the most common occurrence in women. Many women will experience such an episode at some time in their lives. Apart from the distress at the time of the episode, however, an isolated bout of cystitis is not a significant or worrisome medical problem.

Much more important are recurrent symptoms. Recurrent infections can be classified into two categories: *relapse* and *reinfection*.

Relapses

For many women, treatment of their cystitis ends in the disappearance of the discomfort and a presumed "cure." If small numbers of bacteria remain in the bladder, however, symptoms may disappear but the infection may smolder, causing a recurrence of symptoms a few days later. This is a relapse, or persistence of infection. This may occur if antibiotics are stopped before all bacteria have been removed from the bladder. This may also occur in women with kidney stones.

Reinfections

Reinfection is the more common type of recurrent infection, and it happens in more than 80 percent of women who get cystitis over and over again. Bacteria are eliminated and killed, but weeks or months later the woman comes down with another bout of cystitis caused by the same or different bacteria. This is not due to bad or inadequate treatment; it is simply an indication of an especially susceptible urinary tract.

TREATMENT FAILURES

There are also some cases in which treatment will fail because the drugs are simply inadequate for killing the bacteria. In these instances, the urine remains infected with the same organisms. Why does this happen in a day when drug companies are touting "gorrillacillins" that can kill any organism with which they come in contact? Occasionally, the bacteria will be resistant to one of the standard drugs used to treat urinary infection and another drug must be

PAINFUL, FREQUENT URINATION

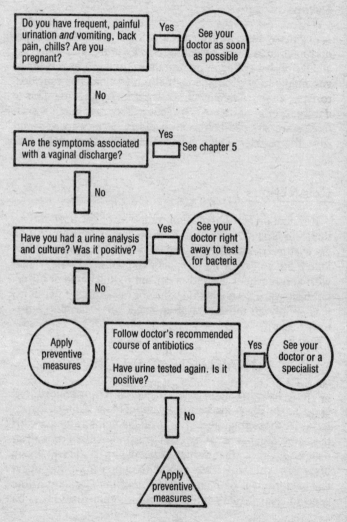

chosen. In other cases, a woman may forget to take the medication on a regular basis or, when she starts feeling better, will simply stop on her own before the drug has had an opportunity to complete its work. (For further information on drugs and their proper use, see Chapters 11 and 12.)

This chart—called a "decision tree" in medical practice—will help you to explain your symptoms clearly to your doctor when you telephone him or her. You may be able to determine right away that it is *not* cystitis and save yourself unnecessary worry, although your doctor may want to examine you anyway. If it is suspicious, you can immediately make an appointment for a urine culture.

KEEP TRACK OF YOUR SYMPTOMS

At the moment when you feel an attack of cystitis coming on, it may be difficult to think of anything except how to get relief fast. Certainly, the things you did or didn't do, ate or drank, or your state of mind, may be blurred in the present experience of pain and the worry about what lies ahead. If you are really serious about discovering what triggers *your* cystitis episodes, I suggest this diary (see chart on next page). Down the left-hand column I have listed the most common triggers in the form of questions that can be answered by a simple "yes" or "no." Across the chart are 28 spaces, one for each day of the month ahead. It makes no difference whether you start in the beginning of a month, in the middle, or at the end, the number of days ahead remain the same. Below the chart are additional spaces to elaborate on your "yes" and "no" answers. For example, if your answer to #7, "Did you change your diet?" is "yes," you may list below just *how* you changed, or what foods were added. I think this chart will be extremely valuable if you are willing to commit yourself to it fully. And even if you do not feel that you have the time to devote to a month's worth, I suggest that you take it out the moment you feel a cystitis attack coming on. It will help to jog your memory as to what transpired in your

| | | **1** | | | | |
	S	M	T	W	Th	
1. Was sexual intercourse more vigorous than usual?						
2. Did you urinate before and after intercourse?						
3. Have you changed your method of birth control?						
4. Did you decrease your fluid intake?						
5. Did you change your usual brand of soap or body cream?						
6. Did you use a feminine hygiene spray or douche?						
7. Did you change your diet?						
8. Did you urinate less often in the last day?						
9. Have you been under unusual stress recently?						
10. Have you worn a pair of tight-fitting hose or slacks?						

life in the prior 24 hours that might be precipitating your symptoms.

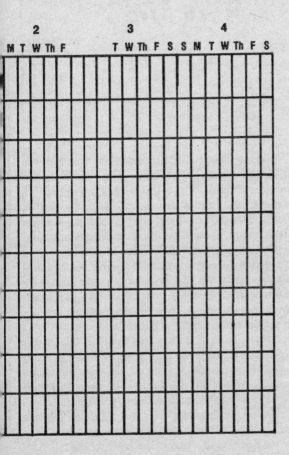

CHAPTER 3

"Why Me?"

The two questions most frequently asked by women who are going through bouts of cystitis are: "Did I catch it from my sexual partner?" and "Why is this happening to me?"

The answer to the first is unreserved: No, you cannot "catch" cystitis from your husband or lover, although as you will soon understand, there are certain conditions in sexual intercourse that make it easier for cystitis to occur.

As for the second question, I wish the answer were as simple. As I explained in the last chapter, cystitis is usually caused by the bacteria called *E. coli*, which live in relative quiet in the lower intestine. Every human—male and female—has a substantial supply of *E. coli* (in addition to other bacteria that make up the intestinal flora). If the simple presence of bacteria were the only causative factor, then everyone would have cystitis or other urinary tract infections all the time. It is only when the bacteria become displaced that trouble begins. The immune system—that intricate network of specialized organs and cells that fights off disease by attacking foreign invaders—is somehow able to distinguish between bacteria in a part of the body where it is normally present (such as *E. coli* in the intestine) and the same bacteria in foreign territory (*E. coli* in the bladder or urethra). In the latter case, the immune system fights the misplaced bacteria just as though it were one that had entered the body from outside.

ROUTES THE *E. COLI* TAKE

How do the *E. coli* become displaced to this foreign territory? Bacteria will thrive wherever it is warm and moist. Consequently, the *perineum* (the skin between the anal opening and the vaginal and urinary opening) becomes a living nursery for opportunistic bacteria. The tissue along the urethra is also an appealing site for bacteria. And, as I explained earlier, the urethra is considerably shorter in women than in men. Thus it is easier for the bacteria to travel up the urethra to the bladder where, in that warm and moist environment, they rapidly multiply.

"Still," you may ask, "why me and not my sister or my best friend?" Science is beginning to answer that question in part with new discoveries about the unique promoting factors in some urinary tracts. The plain fact of the matter is that many women—inadvertently, to be sure—help the bacteria on the journey. *E. coli* are found in vaginal and anal areas. I imagine that many women can still hear their mothers' ringing command: "After you go to the bathroom, wipe yourself from the front toward the back." But wiping from the anus toward the vagina can transport the bacteria-laden stool directly across—and sometimes into—the urethral opening.

Another way in which bacteria are deposited in the urethra is through sexual intercourse. This does not mean that you can "catch" it from your sexual partner; only that the act of intercourse causes pressure along the urethra that pushes bacteria into the bladder. Back in the eleventh century, an Italian physician writing on women's diseases concluded that there was a direct correlation between urinary tract infections and sexual contact. Now, 900 years later, more physicians are confirming that such is the case. In 1977, a study reported that 83 percent of women had their first urinary tract infection after they had become sexually active.

It took a while for Natalie J. to understand that her cystitis was the result of heightened sexual activity and could have happened at any point during her lifetime. Widowed at the age of 49, Natalie soon returned to the financial profession, which she had given up when she married 15 years earlier. When she met Jim, their relationship was, at first, a solid working one, but it soon deepened into a strong physical attraction. After their first night of love-making, Natalie discovered that there was a price to pay for her newly awakened sexual desires. The next day found her with symptoms that were totally unfamiliar: pressure in the lower abdomen, a fierce urgency to urinate, and a burning sensation as the urine flowed through her urethra. By that night, Natalie had developed a slight fever, a headache—and an idea that such intense sexual activity should not be undertaken by someone her age. Her prevention program helped her quickly to dispel that antiquated notion.

When a diaphragm is fitted tightly, as it frequently is, it presses against the bladder. As a result, a diaphragm left in place for up to 8 hours can severely diminish urinary flow and block the easy exit of bacteria. The diaphragm as a foreign body can also change the bacterial balance of the vagina. A recent study showed higher colony counts of *E. coli*, the organism most commonly associated with cystitis, in diaphragm users. This allows more of the bacteria to be present near the urinary opening. The bacteria then need make only a short journey to the urinary tract.

Another possible contributing factor can be certain types of wearing apparel, such as bodysuits, pantyhose, or tight slacks worn for long periods of time. They promote a warm, moist, dark environment, thus increasing the opportunity for bacterial growth.

Another means of bacterial invasion of the bladder, although much less common, is the use of a urinary catheter. The catheter is a long plastic tube that is most commonly used in the hospital during surgery or childbirth to drain the bladder. One study made a few years ago found that nearly half of all hospital-acquired infections are urinary tract infections; more than 90 percent of these are related to genitourinary tract manipulation as in the case of a urinary catheter following surgery.

NATURE CALLS FOR A REASON

In spite of the tenacity of the cystitis-causing *E. coli*, the bacteria gathered at the outside opening of the urethra are usually prevented from entering the urinary tract by the outpouring of urine. In some women, however, the flow of urine is obstructed, or the bladder may not be completely emptied or not emptied frequently enough. The urine in the bladder then becomes a breeding ground for bacteria, which enter the urinary tract unimpeded by the downward flow of urine.

What are the causes of incomplete emptying of the bladder or insufficient urinary output? The obstruction may be caused by a cystocele (a partial herniation of the bladder into the vagina) in the bladder wall, which prevents complete voiding and may lead to stagnation of the remaining urine in the bladder. The obstruction may also be something as simple as a tight-fitting diaphragm which, while it is in place, creates a pressure on the bladder wall, preventing complete emptying. Pregnancy is also a common cause of inefficient emptying of the bladder. Because of the pressure of the growing fetus on the bladder, pregnant women are susceptible to relative stagnation in the urinary system.

By far the most common reason for inefficient emptying of the bladder has less to do with physiological or physical pressures on the bladder than with social and personal pressures—the demands of daily life that prevent many women from adhering to a necessary daily intake of water and other fluids or to a regular and frequent schedule of urination. The amount of liquids you drink determines the amount of urine that is formed. And the amount of urine that is formed is what will be passed out of your body. The bladder's emptying reflex is a defense mechanism that is available to every person. But you need to take the steps to make it work.

CHAPTER 4

Is it Cystitis?
Only Your Doctor
Knows for Sure

The calls usually come early in the morning. "I've been up all night," the voice at the other end of the line says. "I have such a pressure to urinate and then I can't pass more than a trickle. And that little bit burns like hell!" Many times what the woman wants is a call to her local pharmacy for a prescription to cure the attack that she is sure is cystitis.

It certainly would be easy to call in a prescription, especially when all the symptoms are right on target. But the fact is that whether it is a woman's first bout with cystitis, or her one-hundred-and-first, there are certain steps that must be taken to ensure a correct diagnosis.

No matter how classic the symptoms are, no matter how sure both you and your doctor are that it's a full-blown case of cystitis, there are only two ways to be sure: a urine analysis to establish the presence of bacteria and a urine culture to identify the specific organism.

QUESTIONS, QUESTIONS

When a patient comes for a first-time visit, whether the complaint is cystitis or something else, I allow some time for taking a family and personal history. This valuable diagnostic procedure is risk free, involves no super technology, and will take as long as needed to get all the necessary information. The questions are straightforward; some are general and some are specific. My first-time patients are advised to bring along any information they think is relevant with regard to family health history.

The method of history taking varies widely from one doctor to another, and the questions vary, as well. I have selected seven questions—just a random sampling—to give you an idea of what it is that I am looking for and to point out that even the most seemingly far-afield questions may be pertinent to your diagnosis. Obviously, what is important here are not so much the questions but the answers.

1. *Are you married?* It's not that being married per se makes you more or less vulnerable to cystitis, but your answer will give me a first clue to your sexual activity, which may or may not be elaborated upon later in the questionnaire. Cystitis is common to newly married young women as well as in divorced or single women who have stretches of prolonged abstinence that are followed by periods of frequent and vigorous sexual activity.

2. *What is your occupation?* It's not your job responsibilities with which I'm concerned, but how those responsibilities affect your time schedule. Do you allow your work routine to interfere with your normal urge to urinate? Women who attain high-level executive positions sometimes neglect to urinate when first indicated. Not that business women are the only victims of cystitis. I vividly recall a middle-aged woman whose children were grown and were raising families of their own. Had this woman appeared with her symptoms earlier in her life, while she was caring for her children and her home, I might have guessed that her family responsibilities were interfering with her personal habits. The possibility that she might be having an extramari-

tal affair occurred to me, but I quickly discounted that notion when she proceeded to describe how much she and her husband were enjoying their newfound time together. In fact, she went on, they recently had, as a hobby, joined a hiking club. During the long hours on the trails, my patient resisted the urge to urinate, preferring to wait until she was home again. The puzzle was solved.

3. *What is your daily diet?* If I were treating you for high blood pressure, I would suggest reducing your salt intake; if I were treating you for heart disease or obesity, I would suggest cutting down on fatty foods. But what does diet have to do with a bacterial infection? Foods and beverages cannot cause the infection directly, but spicy foods, excessive coffee and tea, and alcoholic beverages tend to irritate a sensitive bladder.

4. *Are you taking any medications?* This is one of the most important considerations in cystitis treatment, which will probably include a course of antibiotics. If you are already taking medicine for any other condition, it is important to make that known. Drugs can interact in a number of ways. Two drugs together can speed up the rate at which either or both are metabolized. Some drugs, when combined, can produce effects that go beyond what one would expect from each drug alone. With such drugs the end result is greater than the sum of the two parts, creating a multiplier effect called potentiation. Furthermore, two drugs together can slow down the rate at which either or both are metabolized. Two drugs interfering with each other in your body can mean that either—or probably both—take much longer to work. Worse, neither may work at all.

When I say "drugs," I include alcohol, one of the most powerful drugs known to society today, as well as "recreational" drugs.

What about vitamins? Many of my patients have read that vitamin C will acidify urine and help prevent infection. Some users have the notion that you can't get enough of a good thing where vitamin C is concerned. Unfortunately, vitamin C in quantities of more than 1 gram a day can lead to toxic effects, including formation of kidney and ureteral stones. Other vitamins can produce unexpected effects as well. For example, a young woman called me in a state of great distress over the fact that her urine had developed a deep yellow discoloration and a strong odor; it took some probing, but what finally came to light was that she had started taking a high-potency vitamin B capsule every morning to try to combat fatigue.

5. *What is your past health history?* During a discussion about medications, the issue of other health problems comes up. Generally, other health problems don't have much effect on whether you will or won't develop cystitis. There are notable exceptions, however. For example, the incidence of urinary tract infection in diabetic women is two to four times greater than in nondiabetic women. There are several reasons for this: an increased glucose in urine, which creates a good medium for bacterial growth; frequent instrumentation of the urinary tract, which makes it more vulnerable to invasion by bacteria; and neurologic lesions, which may affect bladder emptying.

6. *Do you have any allergies?* If you have ever had a reaction to any food, drug, or other substance such as soap or cosmetics, be sure that your doctor knows this. Your symptoms may well be due to an allergic reaction, not an infection. If you are sensitive to drugs such as penicillin, let your doctor know at the start, so that his or her program of treatment does not include penicillin or one of the penicillin-related antibiotics. And try to remember whether you've ever had any bad reaction to a test involving injection of a dye into your bloodstream. Your doctor may want to pursue your symptoms by means of such a test, and your sensitivity

should be on record before you receive it so that you can get some type of medication to prevent an acute allergic reaction.

7. *What are your specific symptoms?* At last, we come to the part you have been waiting for. If you have paid careful attention to Chapter 2, you will be ready with an exacting description of the signs that either will or will not point to cystitis.

THE PHYSICAL EXAM

The next phase of your office visit will move to the examining room where your doctor can perform some important hands-on procedures. By pressing the lower part of your back, on either side of your spine, I can determine the extent of involvement of your kidneys, if any. By pressing gently on your abdomen, I can tell how full of urine your bladder is. If you have told me that you are having a vaginal discharge, I will do an internal vaginal exam and analyze the discharge as well. This is a safeguard against the possibility that the symptoms are due to another disease, or that there are two different diseases going on at one time.

THE SPECIMEN

Although a doctor can often surmise what is wrong with a patient by merely listening to her description of symptoms, for a firm diagnosis it is necessary to examine urine under a microscope—a procedure called urinalysis—and have it cultured in a laboratory.

The way urine is collected can make a difference in the final diagnosis. The key here is "clean catch." There is nothing mysterious about this medical phrase. It simply means that the urine is a perfect specimen of what is inside the bladder, not what is contaminated by organisms lying outside the urinary tract. The first stream of urine will wash away these outside organisms, leaving a stream of urine that represents what is in the bladder.

There is some controversy over *when* urine should be collected for analysis and culture. In most cases, the specimen will be collected in a special glass or plastic container when you arrive in your doctor's office, whether it is early in the morning or late in the day. Many doctors feel that the urine should be collected when you get up in the morning, because it has then had a chance to remain in the bladder for several hours and the offending bacteria will have had a chance to develop. You might, therefore, be asked to collect a urine sample first thing in the morning of the day your appointment is scheduled. The problem with this method, however, is that an overgrowth of bacteria may occur during the interim and the laboratory count will be inflated.

Whenever and wherever you collect your important urine sample, there are fast rules to follow to ensure that it is the best possible representation of what is contained in your bladder.

Before releasing a single drop of urine you should wipe yourself very carefully three times with an antiseptic pad, and repeat the wiping three times, making sure to wipe inside the labia, or lips, around the vaginal opening, and around the anal area. Think of this procedure as sterilizing your genital area. Without such preparation, the urine that passes through your urethra may become contaminated by the surfaces over which it passes.

After carefully cleansing yourself, let a short spurt of urine pass into the toilet. Then begin to collect your urine in the container. And don't feel that it is necessary to fill the cup to the brim; only a small amount is necessary to do the complete urine workup.

PEERING INTO THE WATER

In an article on urinary tract infection in the *FDA Consumer* awhile back, I ran across a wonderful commentary on the historical importance of urine:

FALSTAFF: *What says the doctor to my water?*
PAGE: *He said, sir, the water itself was a good healthy water; but, for the party that owned it, he might have more diseases than he knew . . .*
Henry IV, William Shakespeare

Man has been peering into his water—Shakespeare's word for urine—since time began.* Watercasting (the archaic name for the study of urine) divulged all sorts of things: signs of disease, evil omens, and confirmation of chastity or pregnancy.

The ancient Egyptians, in their medical papyruses, recorded blood in the urine, incontinence or loss of bladder control, burning of the urine, and urgency and frequency of urination. They also utilized what we scornfully refer to as "sewage pharmacology." Fly droppings, feces, gazelle dung, crocodile excrement, mud from burial grounds, and moldy bread were all used for healing purposes. Modern science has recovered penicillin from bread molds, and Aureomycin was originally recovered from soil found near cemeteries.

The formal study of urine began with Hippocrates (460–377 B.C.), that towering figure of early medicine. He believed

---

*In his book, *Urology: A View Through the Retrospectroscope* (Hagerstown, Maryland: Harper & Row, 1973), Dr. John R. Herman, a clinical professor of urology at Albert Einstein College of Medicine in New York City, follows the history of urology and urinalysis from its beginnings.

that the appearance of urine was important to diagnosis of disease and could even give a clue to the expected outcome. He correctly observed that frothy urine was connected with kidney disease.

Uroscopy was the art of looking into a glass container of urine and being able to diagnose the patient's condition and prescribe a course of therapy without necessarily seeing the patient at all. Uroscopy was a natural development of man's curiosity about himself; after all, urine is the most readily examined of the body's outputs.

Urine samples were gathered in a matula for examination. This bulbous clear glass container was divided into four parts, corresponding to the head, breast, stomach, and urinary organs. The changes seen in these parts of the matula identified the location and the nature of the disease.

When uroscopy was at its peak, there were few other diagnostic or clinical testing methods known. Inspection of the urine became more popular and more spectacular, and more of an art than a science. It was done by doctors, uroscopists, watercasters, and even traveling water doctors. These travelers had a good thing going. They would load up with glass matulas and set up a stand in a new village. Customers could take a matula home in its wicker basket and then bring it back filled. The traveling man would examine and diagnose the urine, and prescribe medication that he would then sell. In the next day or so, he moved on to new territory before any results of his diagnosis and therapy became known.

From foretelling or diagnosing pregnancy to predicting the sex of an unborn baby, even the uroscopists and medical doctors often attempted to tell much more than was actually indicated from the urine bubbles, granules, opacities, pus, fat, sand, ash, and other sediment, as well as from the smell, sound, taste, and amount of urine. Often the forecast depended upon what the uroscopist could learn from the messenger who brought the specimen. Many doctors and uroscopists did, however, advance the study of urine. One twelfth-century doctor described 20 different colors of urine and the diseases associated with each. A seventeenth-century London practitioner, Thomas Willis, went one step further. He was the first physician in Europe to note that the urine of diabetic patients was "wonderfully sweet," and he found that out by tasting the urine.

The urine of man or beasts used to be an ingredient in potions and elixirs that claimed to prolong life or restore virility. Black magic used urine in its secret rites, and urine was an important constituent of folk medicines. Ancient Egyptian physicians believed that the urine of a faithful wife cured sore eyes. And it wasn't too long ago that country people used urine as a mouthwash or rubbed it into the gums to relieve toothache.

Modern medicine ascribes no magical powers to urine, but it is as important in helping diagnose some diseases today as it was to ancient doctors. Though urine's appearance and odor still provide valuable clues, nowadays most of the diagnostic action takes place in a laboratory, where urine is examined with the aid of chemicals and a microscope.

The earliest instruments for looking into the genitourinary tract were introduced in the early 1800s. But they all used candles to provide the necessary light, and although some of them were easy to use and actually involved minimal pain, the dangers of working between the legs with lit candles could not be dismissed. Many ingenious devices tried to circumvent the dangers of the candle, but it was not until Thomas Edison invented the incandescent lamp that the closed-off world of the bladder eventually opened up.

THE FIRST STEP: URINALYSIS

The traditional method of performing urinalysis is to spin a few drops of the urine sample in a centrifuge at very high speed. This will separate the sediment from the liquid portion of the urine. Looking at the sediment under a high-powered microscope can reveal what a doctor is searching for right away—white blood cells, which indicate that an infection is underway. The microscopic evaluation may also reveal the presence of red blood cells in the urine even though blood is not detectable to the naked eye.

THE SECOND STEP:
URINE CULTURE

White blood cells and bacteria may be seen in a urinalysis; however, this does not actually identify the bacteria. For this crucial step, a urine culture must be performed in a laboratory. A small amount of urine is inoculated into small containers (such as a petri dish.) Each dish has a different type of culture medium to encourage the growth of bacteria. Bacteria thrive and multiply in these environments. The containers are incubated at 35°C for 24 hours and then examined for bacteria. The count of 100,000 bacteria per milliliter of urine is considered definitive for cystitis, although there are times when a sample from a woman with cystitis will show fewer organisms.

Other tests then are done to identify which specific bacteria are growing in the culture. Different bacteria have different microscopic appearances and chemical properties. Finally, small discs of paper containing antibiotics are placed on a culture of one type of bacteria. If the antibiotic is effective against that particular bacteria, there will be a rim around the paper where the bacteria have been killed.

These urine culture tests take from 48 to 72 hours. If symptoms are significant, treatment should be started immediately with a generally effective antibiotic rather than waiting two to three days for the laboratory results. The antibiotic should be changed if the lab test so indicates. Frequently, if patient can spot the signs of an oncoming cystitis attack, I can schedule an appointment for her at a diagnostic laboratory where her urine can be analyzed and cultured quickly without my having to see her first. Speak to your doctor to determine whether this time-saving process can work for you.

THE THIRD STEP: MORE TESTS

For many of my patients, urinalysis and urine culturing are sufficient. We wait for the results of the urine culture, she follows the prescribed course of antibiotics, and her bout with cystitis is over, never to return or, if it does, not for a long stretch of time.

With a good program of preventive therapy, most women can shield themselves from repeated cystitis attacks. In some cases, however, nothing seems to help: The infections occur over and over again. At this point, with my patient's consent, I will schedule additional uncomplicated tests. Cystitis that does not respond to preventive therapy or antibiotics suggests that something else may be happening in the genitourinary tract, something that might spell danger to the kidneys. Such a possibility should never be left uninvestigated.

What are these additional tests and what do they involve? Here is a brief summary of the ones that I, like your own doctor, might call for:

An *IVP*, intravenous pyelogram, is the simplest kidney x-ray. If some structural abnormality in the urinary tract is causing the recurring infections, this test is likely to show it up. *Pyelo* is the Greek word for the collecting structures that funnel urine from the kidney into the ureter. The intravenous pyelogram is performed by injecting a substance into the bloodstream (usually through a vein in your arm). This substance—a dye—is visible to x-ray and can be rapidly excreted by the kidneys. By taking several x-ray pictures over an hour or so, the collecting structures of the urinary tract can be outlined as the material is excreted. This is an extremely valuable test that often provides the doctor with crucial information. Although the test is very safe, allergic responses can occur if you are sensitive to the dye substance.

The next is *cystoscopy* (see illustration below). A cystoscope, which is much like a miniature periscope on a submarine, is guided into the bladder through the urethra. The

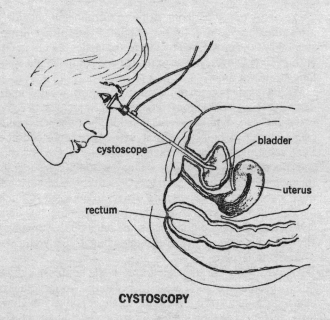

CYSTOSCOPY

instrument makes it possible to look directly into the bladder to locate the openings of the ureters. Minor surgical procedures also can be done through the cystoscope.

A *cystogram* is a test that involves filling the bladder with fluid through a catheter placed in the urethra. Pressure recordings and/or x-rays can be obtained while the bladder contracts and empties.

Not every woman with complicated cystitis will undergo every one of these tests; nor will they necessarily be performed in the same order. In many cases, the tests will be performed only once; in others, the tests may need to be repeated to monitor progress or to pick up complications.

The prospect of these tests may be frightening, but if you are prepared for what will happen, your fears and anxieties should be greatly eased. Here are some questions to ask your doctor and the specialist who may be performing the tests. Be sure that all your questions are answered to your complete understanding before undergoing any tests.

- How is this test going to help diagnose my condition?
- Will the test be done in a doctor's office or in the hospital?
- Will my insurance cover the entire cost of the procedure; if not, how much will be covered?
- What is the exact sequence of steps involved in the test I am about to undergo?
- How long will the test take?
- Will there be any pain or discomfort from this test either during the procedure or following it?
- Am I at special risk for any reason for this particular test?
- Is there anything I should do when I return home after having this test done?
- How long will it take for the results to be reported, and will you call me with the results or should I contact your office?

DO-IT-YOURSELF TESTING: DOES IT REALLY WORK?

It's Friday night of the start of a long holiday weekend. You You have finished your office and housework. Your husband has announced his intention of finally finishing the wood-working project he started months ago. The children have been invited to spend the holiday with friends. There is nothing between you and next Tuesday morning except luxurious hours to do whatever you choose: read, hike, go shopping, go to a museum, give yourself a facial, take a nap, visit with friends. You go to bed early so that you will be bright and full of energy. And suddenly you are awakened by the urgent need to urinate. When you do pass urine, it burns and stings. The pressure in your lower abdomen is noticeable. And the sinking realization sets in that it's about to begin: a bout of cystitis.

Cystitis has a way of arriving at such inopportune moments. Up until several years ago, you would have been left with limited choices: hurry to a hospital emergency room, where urine cultures would be expensive and you might have to spend many hours waiting to see a doctor or trying to contact your own doctor or his or her medical service, which would probably suggest going to an emergency room anyway, or suffer through until the end of the holiday when you might see your doctor.

Recently, there have been a number of home-testing kits made available in drugstores, which promise to indicate the presence of bacteria and the presence of infection. Also, some women may be able to obtain urine cultures from their physician, and perform the preliminary steps themselves, later returning the cultures to the physician for identification of the bacteria.

Any home testing program must be thoroughly discussed with your physician. Bacterial cystitis has too many ramifications to risk the chance that you may misinterpret the reading in any way.

CHAPTER 5

What Else Could It Be?

There are times in medical practice when a consideration of symptoms, plus a physical examination and certain minimal laboratory tests, will positively identify a disease. Like most doctors, I welcome such occasions because it makes life easier for my patient in terms of the diagnostic procedure as well as the early beginning of a course of treatment.

In many cases, however, it is more difficult to pinpoint the cause of symptoms. Certain symptoms may suggest any number of diseases; a headache, for instance, may be caused by eyestrain, stress, allergy, or an underlying neurological disorder. Doctors in search of an answer to their patient's complaints will use what is called differential diagnosis to bring them closer to the solution.

Cystitis is a perfect case in point here. With symptoms such as urgency and frequency in urination, burning, and pains in the lower abdomen, the diagnosis of cystitis would seem clear enough. But what if the urine analysis turns up spotless?

Many of my own patients have turned up such surprises.

Take the case of Claudia, a young woman who had been separated from her husband for nearly a year. During that time, she abstained from sex. "I needed to get my head together," said the now-single mother. But one night she met an attractive man at a local bar and, feeling lonely, allowed him to spend the night with her. About two weeks later, Claudia felt a pain in her abdomen. She had been bicycling a lot, so at first she blamed her discomfort on too much exercise. The pain subsided during her next menstrual period, but afterward it returned, even worse than before. She made an appointment with her doctor who, suspecting a bacterial infection, sent a urine sample off to the laboratory. But the test was negative; the doctor told Claudia that there was little else he could do and that perhaps her new life as a single mother, with all the stresses involved in such a change, was responsible. Claudia's visit (this was in the summer of 1980) coincided with a new report from the New York City Department of Health about a formerly little-known sexually transmitted disease called *Chlamydia*. The incidence of *Chlamydia* had quadrupled in 10 years in New York City; Claudia had become one of the statistics. Fortunately, once *Chlamydia* is diagnosed, it is easy to cure. A two-week course of antibiotics freed Claudia of the infection; she became part of another statistic: women with *Chlamydia* whose infection was cured before it caused permanent damage.

Alice, who had been a patient for many years, also presented a puzzle. Prone to cystitis, Alice had, in recent years, kept that infection under control with a program of prevention. When she appeared one day complaining that urinating was causing a great deal of burning, my first thought was that the problem was a bacterial infection. A number of questions later, however, I had my answer: yeast infection. The clue was the location of the burning; in cystitis it is along the urethra and in a yeast infection the burning is felt on the vulva.

In another case, I recall a patient with very few of the

classic cystitis symptoms, except for intense burning during urination. When her urine sample proved negative, I began to consider other conditions that might be mimicking the cystitis burning. As we spoke, all of my questions seemed to be leading to a void. It was time for another line of questioning, one that frequently turns up surprising answers. I asked my patient if she had changed the brand of any item of personal hygiene. Soap? Personal wipes? Scented toilet paper? Now I was on the right track. My patient had recently purchased a large supply of bubble bath and had been treating herself to long soaks in the bathtub each evening.

I don't mean to suggest that all differential diagnoses are made this easily; in fact, it sometimes takes extensive sleuthing in order to track down the culprit.

CYSTITIS IMITATORS

What are the most common conditions to masquerade as cystitis? What follows is a brief review of the ones that appear with the greatest frequency.

Localized Irritations

Bubble bath brought on the cystitislike symptoms for my patient. Feminine hygiene products, may also cause localized irritation. Even scented toilet paper may cause such problems.

Dietary Triggers

More commonly, the reason for an irritable bladder is dietary: something in whatever is being eaten (or drunk) is reaching the bladder in a form that is highly stimulating both to the bladder lining and the urethra. One of the worst offenders is the all-American favorite, coffee. The villain in coffee, of course, is caffeine, a superpotent stimulant. Caffeine stimulates nearly everything in the body without discrimination— blood pressure, blood vessels, metabolism, gastric secretions, and bladder nerve endings. Decaffeinated brews contain minimal caffeine, but there is still a trace, nonetheless. So very sensitive people would do well to avoid coffee altogether. Not that tea is the answer, either. A brewed tea contains about half the caffeine as a cup of brewed coffee. And to make matters worse for caffeine-sensitive people, there are cola drinks, cocoa, and drugs, both prescription and over-the-counter, filled with the stimulant.

Then there are those foods and drinks that tip the balance of acidity and alkalinity of urine in the bladder. Normally, urine has a pH of 6.8. It can become alkaline if the pH rises to above 7. A pH below 7 means the urine is acid. As the pH becomes more acid it irritates the millions of tiny nerve endings that lie so close to the surface of the bladder. This causes the bladder to respond with increased frequency of urination. The acid pH will also irritate the sensitive membranes of the urethra, resulting in a fairly continuous, dull, burning pain that is likely to intensify during and just after urination.

Another dietary culprit is the spice category—chili peppers and even red and black pepper are likely to stimulate the bladder and urethra. These do not cause infection but may bring on symptoms of bladder irritation. But few people use such spices day in and day out. (In Chapter 10, you will find a list of foods, beverages, and spices, to avoid when you design your personal cystitis prevention plan.)

Irritation can occur during sexual intercourse by a diaphragm creating friction against the bladder.

OTHER DISEASES IMITATING CYSTITIS

These cystitis masqueraders are fairly simple to pinpoint; a highly spiced meal or a high intake of caffeine in beverages or medicines that bring on symptoms in full force are highly suggestive of a cause and effect. Unfortunately, it is not always so simple to unmask the pretender. Here are a few of the underlying physical conditions that I would look for in the absence of bacteria in the urine:

Endometriosis

This condition is caused by the growth of tissue similar to the tissue lining the uterus (or endometrium) beyond the uterine walls. These endometriotic cells form patches and scars throughout the pelvis and around the ovaries and fallopian tubes, resulting in a variety of symptoms, the most common of which is pain. In some cases, endometriotic implants can be found on the bladder, or parts of the intestine.

The diagnosis is usually made by laparoscopy, a procedure in which a laparoscope is inserted into the abdomen, usually at the belly button, and the physician looks into the pelvis for characteristic implants.

Endometriosis regresses during pregnancy and menopause. Traditional treatment attempts to mimic pregnancy with administration of progesterone or estrogen and progesterone given in sufficient dosage to stop menstrual periods. The side effects, including bloating, nausea, and breast discomfort were unpleasant for many women. Danocrine, a relatively new drug and antiestrogenic agent, approximates menopause, another time when endometriosis is known to regress. Side effects may include hot flashes, vaginal dryness, and some male hormone effects, including deepened voice and hair growth. If endometriotic implants are extensive or large, then surgery or surgery and drug therapy together may be required.

Stress Incontinence

Urinary incontinence is the involuntary loss of urine. There are several different types of incontinence, the most common of which is *stress incontinence*. A weakening of the bladder and pelvic floor muscles may occur after childbirth, especially after a difficult delivery or delivery of a large child. Hereditary factors are also important.

Stress incontinence is less common in some populations than others. For example, the condition is less common in black women than in Caucasian women. The symptoms of stress incontinence frequently become apparent after menopause, when changing hormone levels affect tissue tone. Any additional stress—caused by sneezing, coughing, laughing, or other exertion—can result in leakage of small amounts of urine.

Urge Incontinence

Urge incontinence is characterized by a sudden, uncontrollable urge to urinate that cannot be restrained. If a toilet can be reached immediately, loss of urine may occur.

Overflow Incontinence

This is characterized by small amounts of urine that leak out when the bladder is full. Frequently the sensation of the bladder being full has been lost. This may occur temporarily when the bladder is overdistended, after surgery or childbirth, or occasionally with a primary attack of herpes, which has affected the nerves of the bladder. It may occur chronically in some cases, with permanent nerve damage secondary to spinal cord injuries, diabetes, or neurological diseases such as multiple sclerosis.

Incontinence Testing

A woman who experiences incontinence for the first time should be tested for urinary tract infection (UTI). If UTI is not present, then urodynamic or cystometric testing is warranted. In these procedures, the bladder is filled with fluid or gas, and pressure measurements taken. Depending on the type of incontinence, it may be treated with urinary antispasmodics or surgery.

Gonorrhea

Gonorrhea is a sexually transmitted disease. Although the symptoms vary, they sometimes include a sudden increase in frequency and urgency of urination, occasionally accompanied by pain, causing patients to suspect a UTI. Some women experience discharge and/or burning (these symptoms are more common in men). Gonorrhea is frequently asymptomatic in women. If you have gonorrhea, both you and your sexual partner must be treated. Treatment may be antibiotics taken orally, or by injection. A second culture should be done a week following treatment to insure that the bacteria have been completely destroyed.

Genital Herpes

This is also a sexually transmitted disease, but it is caused by a virus called the herpes simplex virus. The first symptoms in a primary herpes attack may be irritation or itching in the genital area. Blisters form in the genital area; these are very painful and often the pain is sensed in other nearby areas, such as the bladder or the urethra. The blisters break quickly, however, and leave raw, ulcerated areas. Because painful and difficult urination may occur from urine passing over raw areas and from the herpes virus attacking nerves in the area, patients often call the doctor thinking that they have UTI.

Recurrent herpes attacks are much less painful than the primary attack. In these, there is usually only a single lesion, frequently accompanied by a bladder sensation such as tingling or hesitation during urination. Zovirax, orally or as a topical ointment, is used to treat primary attacks of herpes. In some women with frequent recurrences, a long-term prophylactic regimen of Zovirax may be given. Women with infrequent reoccurrences may find local treatment sufficient.

Chlamydia

Caused by an intracellular parasite, this is probably the most elusive of all the sexually transmitted diseases. The organisms are difficult to culture and the symptoms closely mimic many other disorders. *Chlamydia* is frequently asymptomatic. Symptoms may include discharge and a vague burning sensation on urination. *Chlamydia* is hard to culture because it is an intracellular parasite and culture results may require up to two weeks.

Recently, two new tests were developed using monoclonal antibodies to detect the presence of *Chlamydia*. With these tests, results are now available within days, instead of weeks, and treatment can be started quickly. Treatment is simple once the *early* detection is made and consists of at least two weeks of antibiotics for the woman and her sex partner. Retesting must be done after treatment has been completed. Left untreated, *Chlamydia* may lead to pelvic inflammatory disease (or PID) (see below), ectopic pregnancy, and infertility.

Nonspecific Urethritis (NSU)

NSU is a name traditionally used for urethritis in men that was not gonorrhea. Less commonly, the term was used for women with similar symptoms. We know that many of these infections were caused by *Chlamydia* or *Mycoplasma*. *Mycoplasma* is an organism similar to *Chlamydia*, but its role in causing PID or infertility is more in doubt than that of *Chlamydia*. Treatment is similar to that for *Chlamydia*.

Pelvic Inflammatory Disease (PID)

PID is an inflammation in the pelvic organs, that is, the uterus, fallopian tubes, and ovaries. It may be caused by a gonorrhea or *Chlamydia* infection. Once it starts, frequently other bacteria become involved. Minor cases may be treated with oral antibiotics; more serious cases require hospitalization and intravenous antibiotic therapy. Treatment must begin promptly to avoid damage to the fallopian tubes.

Monilial Infection

Monilial infections, also known as fungus or yeast infections, are caused by a microorganism called *Candida albicans*. A small amount of *Candida* is always present in the body and, occasionally, when homeostasis is out of balance in a certain area, the condition may grow uncontrollably, causing the symptoms of a yeast infection. Precipitating factors may include use of antibiotics, dietary changes (especially increases of sugar), birth control pills, or pregnancy. The latter two change the hormone balance of the vagina in a way that favors yeast growth. Certain women are more susceptible than others to monilial infections. Symptoms include thick, cottage cheeselike discharge, itching and burning of the vulva. Sex may be painful and burning may occur during urination. Diagnosis can be made by examining a smear of the secretion under a microscope or doing a culture. Treatment is usually a vaginal cream or suppository. Monilia-prone women may need to use suppositories preventively during antibiotic use. Live-culture yogurt placed directly in the vagina may also be useful in treating monilial infections.

Trichomoniasis

This is a common type of vaginitis caused by a single-cell parasite called *Trichomonas vaginalis*. The symptoms include discharge and burning. If the vagina and vulva are very irritated, urination may be painful. Trichomoniasis is diagnosed by examination of the discharge on a microscopic slide in the doctor's office. An antibiotic called metronidazole is used for treatment. The male sex partner must also undergo treatment. Although men usually exhibit no symptoms, if the male partner is not treated, he will act as a reservoir for the organism and reinfect the woman.

Prolapsed Bladder

After childbirth, especially if the delivery is difficult and the baby is large, the pelvic floor muscles may be weakened. Genetic factors also play a role in some families. Kegel exercises (forced tightening and relaxation of the perinaal muscles) will help tone them after childbirth. After menopause, with the dropping of hormone levels, the tissues in this area are weakened further and some women may experience a dropping down or falling out of the pelvic organs, which may create a pressure sensation. It may also interfere with the complete emptying of the bladder. A prolapsed bladder *can* be a cause of cystitis because it prevents complete emptying of the bladder. Some women learn how to replace their bladder manually during urination. An alternative to manual replacement is the installation of a pessary (a hard rubber ring) into the vagina to support the bladder. Surgery may also be performed to reinstate the bladder to its proper position.

Fibroids

These lumps of fibrous tissue grow in the muscle wall of the uterus, usually in women over 30. Depending on size and position, fibroids can cause bladder pressure and a feeling of fullness, which interferes with urination.

CHAPTER 6

Complications of Cystitis

We are acutely aware of the importance of minutes in certain medical situations: heart attack, bleeding, choking, gunshot wounds, stabbings, automobile accidents. These are the stuff of television drama, and when they happen in real life, our instinct tells us to move as quickly as possible.

I believe that the same rapid reflex behavior should be applied when a woman starts to experience urgency and frequency in urination, burning urine, pain in the lower abdomen—symptoms that eventually might be diagnosed as bacterial cystitis. I cannot emphasize too much the importance of early treatment of the infection once it starts—not only for the best chances of curing the disease, but to avoid the complications that can develop if cystitis is not treated or is treated too late. In the following pages, I will summarize some of the more common complications of untreated cystitis.

WHAT CAN HAPPEN IF YOU DON'T GET MEDICAL HELP

After reading, you will have at your disposal every means to circumvent the bacterial infection.

Cystitis Cystica

This condition is characterized by small bacteria-filled cysts in the bladder lining. Symptoms of the condition are identical to those for simple cystitis, but they can disappear and recur periodically over months and years.

Acute Pyelonephritis

This is an infection in the kidney. It may have begun as a bladder infection which, uncontrolled, traveled to the kidneys, or it may have reached the kidneys via the bloodstream. The symptoms may include chill accompanied by a high fever, pain in the lower back just above the waist, shaking, and teeth chattering. The pain may continue down into the groin area, and joints and muscles may also ache. There is little urinary frequency or urgency here as with bladder infections. The pain tends to be continuous and does not come in waves as it might with other kidney diseases; it stays in one spot and is worsened by moving around. The infection is confirmed by means of a urine culture. It is very important that the exact identification be made so that the proper drug can be used in a course of treatment.

Chronic Pyelonephritis

If infections in the urinary tract continue over a number of years, they can cause kidney damage. Though rare today, if untreated, chronic pyelonephritis could lead to kidney failure.

Hypertension

This is commonly known as high blood pressure and may be the result of long-term kidney disease. The kidneys manufacture and release special chemicals that maintain normal blood pressure levels. An infection running rampant may interfere with this precise system, upsetting the routes of the chemical messengers. Salt and water may then be retained by the body, which in turn increases the volume of plasma in the blood, raising blood pressure.

Pregnancy Problems

During pregnancy, hormonal changes cause a general relaxation in the muscle tone of the urinary system, resulting in retention of urine in the ureters and bladder. Also, symptoms of urinary tract infections may be hard to differentiate from the symptoms of pregnancy because both may cause urinary pressure and frequency. Many studies have shown that women who develop urinary tract infections during pregnancy have an increased risk of premature labor or delivery. Women who have had a history of UTI should be tested during pregnancy and promptly treated with antibiotics if infection occurs. The choice of antibiotics is limited, in order to use only drugs that are safe for mother and fetus. In any event, the side effects of an untreated UTI can be far more serious than the side effects of a properly chosen antiobiotic during pregnancy. (For a detailed discussion of cystitis in pregnancy, see Chapter 13.)

PART II

OVERCOMING CYSTITIS

CHAPTER 7

Is Your Doctor Good for You?

We all work hard at our personal relationships—with our spouses, children, other relatives, friends, the people we work with. The result is a special bond that develops between us and the other person, a bond that can be strengthened by each encounter. Sometimes even the process of building the relationship is its own reward.

I think a woman's relationship with her doctor merits the kind of consideration that is extended to other relationships in life. How do you choose a doctor who can guide you through illness and encourage you to health? Several of the conventional ways to find a good physician that have come down through time—asking friends, checking credentials, and calling the local medical society—are no guarantee that you will find a doctor who is good for *you*. What you should be looking for is a doctor who combines the best virtues of training and personality; a search, I admit, that may be easier said than done.

This is not to dismiss recommendations of friends, and co-workers. This is not exactly a scientific way of going about finding a doctor, but it works for many people. The trick is not to ask if the other person "likes" the doctor—tastes, preferences, and needs may be very different—but to ask specific questions about the doctor's practice and approach to diagnosis and treatment.

The most important piece of advice I can give you here is: *Choose a doctor when you are healthy.* When you are sick and anxious, perhaps in pain and maybe even running a high fever, you should not have to start shopping around for a doctor. I suggest that you consider a primary care physician rather than a medical specialist who will treat only specific disorders. If it turns out that you do need a specialist, this primary care physician is in the best position to make a good referral.

Here are some points worth considering:

- *How accessible is the doctor?* It should be fairly easy for you to get to the doctor's office from your home or place of work. Accessibility also includes the doctor's hours; you should look for someone whose hours will allow for you to make appointments without too much alteration in your daily schedule.

- *What about fees?* If a doctor's fees are too high, you are likely to put off making an appointment unless you are in the most dire circumstances. Be sure your doctor's fees are in line with your own income, and settle *all* matters having to do with insurance coverage before you go in for your first visit. Most doctors will want to be paid at the time of the visit or shortly thereafter, but should gladly help you fill out the necessary insurance claim forms. If a doctor's fees are beyond your means, ask for a referral.

- *Does the sex of the doctor matter?* Probably not as much as some people think, or at least not in ways that we would be led to believe. It is entirely possible to find women who are as aloof as men are reported to be and, on the other hand, men who are as empathetic and considerate as women are expected to be. Women do have

• an edge with gynecological areas only because they may have suffered through the very diseases and conditions for which you are seeking help. As far as age goes, I believe that it makes less difference how old a doctor has grown than whether he has stopped growing. Continuing medical education in this day is not just a good thing to do, but an essential ingredient in the practice of excellent medicine.

• *Does the doctor's staff seem efficient and courteous?* Some offices fairly hum with an air of efficiency, staff is busy but there is a kind of positive electricity in the air that is obvious to anyone who is in the waiting room. In some cases, this translates to frenzy, with staff scurrying about with wasted motions, telephones ringing constantly and a general stressful atmosphere. An overworked staff member cannot be expected to be courteous to a patient, not if a few extra seconds of conversation will mean that her work will go undone or that she will have to stay late to complete it. Your doctor's staff is an important part of your health care.

• *Does the doctor talk in your language?* Earlier in this book, I suggested that you try to avoid phrases such as "down there," "you know where," and "number 1." On the other hand, I wish that all doctors, no matter what their specialty, would avoid using language that only another medical person can understand. It won't mean much to you to know that there are over 100,000 microorganisms per milliliter of your urine unless you have some frame of reference, the most important of which is that this is *my* frame of reference for infection. I was impressed with the attitude of one of my patients, a journalist, who followed each of my statements by her own question, "What do you mean by that?" She explained that it was partly habit from her years of interviewing doctors to get them to describe and explain what they were talking about so that she could offer the information to readers. It worked so well, she said, that she used the interview format in her own experiences and never came away from a doctor's visit confused.

- *Does the doctor pay attention to you?* If you find yourself cut off in midsentence or, worse, not being able to squeeze a word in edgewise at all, something is amiss in this doctor/patient relationship. To me, conversation is as important a part of a patient visit as the physical examination. Although my time is often limited, I try to reserve a few minutes to hear a patient's response to my question, "How are you doing?" Recently, this was brought home to me with Laura, a young law student who returned to the college health service again and again with cystitis-related symptoms. Nothing seemed to help her and I suspect they were looking for the wrong clues. After a conversation with Laura about her career and her studies, I quickly recognized a fellow overachiever and suggested that she cut down on the factors that were causing stress in her life. Laura's immediate decision was to drop one of the courses that crammed her schedule. Shortly afterward, she wrote to me to say that her symptoms had disappeared.

- *Does the doctor care about what you eat?* I don't claim that eating certain foods and excluding others is going to cure your cystitis or any other disease, for that matter. Foods do play an important role in this disease, but not without all the other factors used in a preventive program. The importance of a sound diet goes far beyond single diseases to the state of the whole person. I care very much about what you eat on a day-to-day basis, because it gives me a very good idea about how you will respond to the therapy set up in a prevention/ treatment program.

- *Does the doctor have nonoffice-hour availability or provision for attention?* One of my patients told me, half in jest, that all of her cystitis attacks happened at 9 o'clock on Friday night of a holiday weekend. In other words, they all happened when I was somewhere other than in my office. But someone is always available for me when I am not; the covering doctors are all qualified to do exactly what I would do in the emergency situation.

- *Does your doctor allow you to bring another person along?* I think that having a friend or spouse along on an office visit, especially the first one, can be helpful and reassuring for a patient. I am not saying that women are incapable of handling situations like this on their own, or that they are incapable of understanding what the doctor is saying without an interpreter. All I am saying is that a person in discomfort or pain is not as likely to hear everything that is being said. If another person accompanies you on an office visit and examination, give them a pen and paper to take notes.

- *Does your doctor make your medical records available?* Any patient who is treated by more than one physician should obtain and keep copies of outside laboratory records so that these will not be duplicated. Alternately, have your physician send copies of your test results to your other physicians.

- *Does your doctor accept/encourage a second opinion?* A secure and confident patient is one who is most likely to participate in her own recovery. If her confidence comes from having my diagnosis confirmed, so much the better. And if my diagnosis might be improved, so much the better, too. Certainly, I would encourage a second opinion when any radical procedure is indicated, for example, surgery or experimental drugs. I would also encourage a second opinion if, after a considerable period of time, I feel that I have exhausted all of my diagnostic options and the patient is still having symptoms.

CHAPTER 8

Making Habits Work for You

"I'm so in the habit of letting cystitis rule my life that I find I'm a little frightened now that I probably won't have to cope with it anymore."

Joan S., one of the women who entered the cystitis prevention program in its infancy, brought the problem of habits home to me with that comment. An office manager for a large construction firm, Joan once weighed 40 pounds more than her acceptable weight, smoked two packs of cigarettes a day, and rarely exercised. One day, she looked at herself in the mirror and announced that her days of sloth were over. She embarked upon a plan of eating that emphasized a change in behavior, knowing that she would never stick to a traditional diet. Then, she smoked what she had decided was her last cigarette, and went cold turkey. What's more, she is now, six months after this revelation, running 3 miles a day and feeling wonderful.

With all of the conscious and successful effort that went into these remarkable alterations, one would assume that Joan would have no problem making the small changes in her lifestyle that would free her from her regular cystitis attacks, or at least reduce their frequency. But time and again

Joan would come in for testing and, upon identification of the bacteria, treatment with antibiotics. Each time she would admit that she had, indeed, brought on the infection herself by lapsing in the protective patterns she had promised to carry out. "I start out for a day or two drinking a lot of water and making regular bathroom trips. Then I get busy and all caught up in the office routines and everything you told me was forgotten," she explained. "It's almost as though I've accepted this disease as part of my life."

In my experience with cystitis patients, I've realized that in many ways habits are more tenacious than the bacteria that breed in the bladder. Thinking rarely enters into the patterns that are built around habits. These patterns of behavior seem to happen automatically, as though they were part of the nervous system that controls involuntary body activities. An old Czechoslovakian proverb tells us that a habit is a shirt made of iron. For anyone who has been bound by that inflexible restraint, there often seems to be no way out.

I realized long ago that I could go on and on telling women about their bad habits, and even their good ones. But until *each woman* made a prevention a part of *her own* life, I would be wasting my breath. I would continue being a crises-oriented body mechanic, a repair person rather than someone who could prevent the breakdowns in the first place. My patients, I decided, had to tell *me* how they were going to break *their* habits. They had to become activists, rather than passive objects of my repair work. So I developed a habit-breaking plan that could be applied to any negative habit at all.

The plan will work for you as it has for many of my cystitis patients who try to shed their "iron shirt." Breaking out of long-standing patterns is never easy, and the likelihood of slipping back is always present. But perseverance pays off.

BREAKING HABITS BY H-A-B-I-T

H stands for headwork, the mental energy you will apply to breaking your harmful habits.

A stands for approval, and by this I mean the decision that you don't have to settle for sickness, that you deserve to be well.

B stands for behavior, including the changes you will consciously make.

I stands for information, all the facts and facets of cystitis that you are gathering from this book.

T stands for thoughts, your statements to yourself that confirm your determination and, indeed, your success.

Before going on, it is important that you understand three things: your goal, the interrelatedness of the H-A-B-I-T elements, and your acceptance of responsibility.

The goal, certainly, is preventing cystitis. But as you work toward this end you will find that you are achieving something more: a sense of control over not only this condition but also other aspects of your life.

The interrelation of the H-A-B-I-T elements is an important point to grasp, because none of them will work as well in isolation as they will together. They reinforce and complement one another. In fact, there is probably a synergistic effect: When all the elements are working in perfect unison, the whole becomes greater than the sum of the parts. Don't approach the formula selectively. For example, don't decide to work on behavioral changes to the exclusion of all the other elements. For one thing, it won't work that way; what's more, you could be overlooking an element that is even more important to your well-being.

Finally, the nucleus of control in this formula is right where *you* are. *You* make the decisions, *you* make the changes, and *you* reap the rewards. You will gain as much as you give to the process, so give it your all.

H: Headwork

Over and over again, a woman will say to me, "I'll do anything to be rid of this terrible disease." I listen very carefully to this kind of statement, because sometimes I can hear much more than mere words. When I hear a tone of voice that announces anxiety, fear, resentment, anger, or embarrassment, I know that I am listening to a person who has accepted the role of victim.

Rarely do all of the negative feelings surface in the way they did in Stephanie K., a flight attendant whose first attack of cystitis happened while she was in Italy. Treated with antibiotic therapy there, her infection subsided, only to reemerge while she was in Paris. By the time Stephanie went in for treatment she was distraught. "It's ruining me, ruining me," she said repeatedly. Her doctor tried to assure her that because the infection had been caught early enough both times, the chance that any permanent damage had been done was small. A dedicated program of preventive therapy that would probably reduce her attacks or maybe end them completely was prescribed. This did not reassure Stephanie at all. It finally was revealed that the pilot with whom she usually flew on those overseas trips had become her lover—a fact that she had kept secret from her steady boyfriend in New York. Now the jig was up, she thought, because, as she put it, "Everybody knows that you get cystitis from sexual excesses." Stephanie had to be assured that although the infection might have been brought on by sexual activity, there could have been other factors, as well. Her doctor further suggested that she view her cystitis for what it really was: an infection caused by a bacteria, capable of causing *only* an infection, not the breakup of a romance. She was not convinced; her attitude of defenseless victim was complicating her condition more than she could ever realize.

It might be stretching it to say that Stephanie ever considered her cystitis a mixed blessing, but she did eventually come to terms with her feelings about the two men in her life. Her New York boyfriend, it seems, wanted to hear none of the facts about cystitis that Stephanie came home with after her first office visit. His accusations continued for several days, until finally Stephanie insisted that he move out of her apartment. It was a relief although she was deeply hurt over the fact that someone would impede her attempts at recovery. "It was almost as though he enjoyed seeing me suffer. I deserve better than that!"

Scientists are not quite ready to say that you can think your way to good health, but studies are providing tangible evidence for a connection between emotions and disease. Just 10 years ago, textbooks and researchers portrayed infection, for instance, as the simple, predictable outcome of a disease-causing microbe encountering a susceptible host. Various factors such as old age, malnutrition, and fatigue could make a disease more severe. But there was surely no room for the fanciful notion that elation, depression, anxiety, anger, fear, contentment, or stress could affect the course of a disease.

Today, that wisdom is being revised by scientists around the world whose work in laboratories with animals and humans has identified specific ways in which stress can affect the body's immune defenses against disease. Once upon a time, such investigations were called folklore; today they are called psychoneuroimmunology, or behavioral immunology. The basic theme is that cellular changes caused by any negative emotions can have physical effects on the body's defenses. How does this happen? The theory centers on the body's first line of defense of the immune system: the white blood cells, called lymphocytes. These include

B cells, which manufacture antibodies against microbes; helper T cells, which aid the B cells in making the right kind of antibodies; and killer T cells, which wipe out invading organisms if they have been exposed to them before. Together with scavenger white blood cells that gobble up dead cells and debris, the various types of lymphocytes work in coordination to police the body's tissues.

The initial studies in this growing field showed that the lymphocyte response was depressed—sometimes severely—when a patient was under stress. Recently, studies have been showing something even more interesting: It is not so much the stress that causes depression of the immune system, but rather an individual's feeling of being out of control of a stressful situation. In one experiment, behavioral immunologist Mark Laudenslager and his colleagues at the University of Denver gave mild electric shocks to 24 rats. Half the animals could switch off the current by turning a wheel in their enclosure, whereas the other half could not. The rats in the two groups were paired so that each time one rat turned the wheel it protected both itself and its helpless partner from the shock. Laudenslager found that the immune system was depressed below normal in the helpless rats but not in those that could turn off the electricity.

In people, studies bear out the same findings. For example, a study of women with breast cancer found that those who reacted with anger and determination to beat the disease were more likely to be alive 10 years later than those who gave in to it.

The mechanisms that account for the connection between the mind and the immune system are still under intense study, but it has been found that anxiety triggers the release of many hormones that provide the answers. Stress also stimulates secretion of chemicals called neuropeptides, which influence mood and emotions.

Eventually, researchers will be able to pinpoint the benefits to health of positive emotions of hope, affection, love, mirth, joy, and self-approval. This brings us to the next step in the formula.

A: Approval

Toilet training is an important part of our culture. Even as small children we learn the importance of being able to "hold it" until we get to a convenient bathroom. Much of our early self-confidence is built upon achievements like this, and throughout our lives, we carry the sense of self-control, a feeling of pride that we are not subject to the whims of our involuntary muscles.

Cystitis changes all that. An attack of cystitis, with the two major symptoms—urgency and frequency—can plunge a woman into the lowest depths of self-deprecation and even guilt. One of my patients even spoke of her recurring cystitis as the primary reason for divorce.

Ellen W., a 30-year-old teacher, had been married for three years when her cystitis attacks began. Her husband, who worked in Washington D.C., lived in that city during the week, and commuted back to New York on the weekends. Every Monday morning, after a weekend of lovemaking, Ellen found herself with the beginnings of an attack. Soon she began to dread the weekends, an attitude that became very apparent to her husband. Some weekends passed without his making the trip home, which bothered Ellen because she felt lonely without him. But she also felt relieved, because she knew that during the week ahead she would be free of the symptoms. Eventually, the marriage ended. In the months after the divorce, Ellen realized that the marriage had been on shaky ground to begin with, and the cystitis was not the cause but only a trigger for the breakup. But that didn't make it any easier for her to regain her self-esteem. "Unclean," was the word that she used repeatedly to describe herself when she came in for treatment. Ironically, her cystitis attacks continued after the divorce, indicating that it was not *only* sexual relations that brought on the infection. Ellen, at one point, asked: "Why do I feel that my femininity has been compromised by this disease?" Telling her not to feel that way was futile. There had to be a better way to help Ellen regain her approval of herself.

When Ellen came to me for treatment, I suggested that she make a list of those attributes that made her feel particularly good about herself. I reminded her that she had special training that qualified her to educate small children, that she had special skills in quiltmaking that had enabled her to design and make quilts to order, and that she also must have some tricks in the art of living that enabled her to maintain a high energy level (when she wasn't having a cystitis attack).

Ellen began to think about these personal gifts and to see them as positive qualities that were *right* with her instead of negative and wrong.

At first glance, the qualities that Ellen began to see in herself seemed small and insignificant to her. But upon closer examination, they proved that little things do mean a lot. Like Ellen, we all have certain skills and abilities that help us refresh ourselves, to restore our energy for useful work or play; ways in which we are able to introduce some tranquility into our lives; ways to stretch our mind and even our body beyond its current limits. Seeing herself in a more objective fashion helped Ellen to understand that real health is more than just an absence of symptoms, it is a dynamic process. "I need to conquer this disease," she finally said to me one day. "I am ready to give it all I've got—although I'm not quite sure what 'it' is."

B: Behavior Changes

Perhaps you're not even aware that some of the things you are doing as a matter of course are causing or at least contributing to your cystitis attacks. Let's take a minute to review some of the illness-inviting habits that may be resulting in misery.

Bad Habit #1. Insufficient water intake. Even under normal circumstances, people should drink eight glasses of water a day to keep things moving in the genitourinary system. For a cystitis sufferer, the daily quotient should be even higher. The constant passage of water through the bladder does two things: It flushes the bacteria out of the bladder where they have begun to breed, and it dilutes the urine, making it less hospitable to bacteria seeking a place to grow. Water is contained in many beverages and foods that are usually consumed on a daily basis (see Chapter 10 for a complete listing). But for the best results, nothing beats a glass of straight water.

Bad Habit #2. Infrequent and/or incomplete urination. Urine is normally sterile, that is, it contains no bacteria and no built-in defense mechanisms. Therefore, bacteria can have a field day once they enter the bladder where urine is waiting to be excreted. The entire burden of preventing bacterial growth depends on the voiding mechanism which, when it works frequently and completely, can wash out entire populations of bacteria. When urine is retained in the bladder for longer than 3 hours, or when urinating does not empty the bladder completely, the bacteria continue to multiply at an incredibly rapid rate.

Bad Habit #3. Careless hygiene. I doubt that there are many women who have not heard, at some point during their early toilet-training years, "Wipe yourself from front to back." I can hardly imagine that our mothers were sophisticated enough in medicine to know that, following a bowel movement, bacteria remained in the fecal matter at the anal opening. But they knew that the area was unclean and, therefore, should not be wiped across the nearby openings to the vagina and urethra. Now we *know* that bacteria lurk near the anal opening. *Always*—not sometimes or most of the time—wipe yourself from the front to back.

Bad Habit #4. Tight-fitting clothes. Tight jeans and control-top pantyhose do not allow for air circulation around the genital area. This encourages a warm, moist environment—just what bacteria love. The same holds true for synthetic undergarments. Choose clothing carefully. Cotton undergarments are best; second best are those with a cotton crotch.

Bad Habit #5. Infrequently changed sanitary napkins. A sanitary napkin, or a tampon, moistened with blood and lying close to your urethral opening, is another fine culture medium for bacteria. Both forms of feminine protection must be changed every 4 to 6 hours to ensure that bacteria do not have any opportunity to multiply.

Bad Habit #6. Retaining urine before/after intercourse. This is thoroughly covered in the following chapter. For now, remember that pressure along the urethra during intercourse will help to move bacteria from the vaginal area into the urethra. If there is a residue of urine in the bladder before intercourse, and if it is not eliminated immediately afterward, the bacteria will quickly multiply.

Bad Habit #7. Wrong food choices. This is not to say that a poor diet or even eating the wrong kinds of foods can cause cystitis, just that the urine produced as a result of these factors can encourage the growth of bacteria. (Chapter 10 details the foods to focus on or avoid.) Even if your cystitis symptoms are not a result of bacterial infection, some foods can bring on irritable bladder and urethra problems.

I: Information

Cystitis has not been a taboo subject like rape and incest, but neither has it been astonishing, like heart transplants or attachment of severed limbs. Consequently, it has received little attention in magazines or newspapers read by the general public. Unfortunately, in the void that should have been filled by good solid facts, myths and misinformation have abounded.

It is rare to find a patient with recurrent cystitis who isn't toting about some excess mythological baggage concerning the disease. This results in a weighty burden that only impedes recovery and self-help. In the first part of this book, I have provided every fact you need to know about cystitis—its causes, confusions, complications. I think that a thorough reading of this material will help put the infection in perspective for you. Remember, cystitis is an infection, not a moral failure on your part. I hope that you are curious enough to refer back to the first six chapters often—and to pass along the information to others who could benefit from it.

Josh Billings, the nineteenth-century writer and observer of human life, once observed, "It is better to know nothing than to know what ain't so." Cystitis is a good case in point: With wrong information, sufferers will eagerly try any unproven cure or, worse, accept the disease as their lot in life. With knowledge, you begin to look at your situation from a different point of view, from the perimeter rather than the center, where it is almost aways impossible to recognize anything except the dire situation you are in. Objectivity is the key to overcoming cystitis, because it enables you to deal successfully with the negative physical and emotional aspects of your disease, and enhance your body's capacity to thwart it.

T: Thoughts

History tells us that the man who built the Bastille was later imprisoned in it. The carpenter who built Boston's first set of stocks was accused of overcharging for the job and became its first prisoner. A rigid ecclesiastic invented the iron cage, a torture chamber constructed so that the victim could neither stand upright or lie down in it. The inventor himself later spent 11 years in his own invention.

Cystitis sufferers, too, are confined in prisons of their own making, caught in traps they have laid with their thoughts about themselves. What kind of pattern is dominant in your thoughts and emotions? Let's take a look at the ways you view yourself. Here are a dozen statements that I have heard over and over again from women who suffer from chronic, recurring cystitis attacks:

"I'll never lead a normal life."
"I'll never be able to enjoy sex."
"I think I am being punished for having sex."
"I am sure I will contaminate my lover."
"I don't want to leave the house."
"There's nothing like cystitis to ruin a career."
"I get headaches from the tension."
"I must have been born with this disease."
"I'm sure it is causing permanent damage."
"Why doesn't medicine have a cure for this?"
"I'm afraid of getting pregnant."
"Why me?"

All of us constantly engage in self-talk, internal thought language that describes and interprets the world around us.

The preceding self-talk is self-deprecating and self-limiting: It creates impossible barriers to healthy living.

How can such thoughts be stopped? By conscious effort. It's simple, but not easy.

Thought-stopping involves concentrating on the negative thoughts and, after a brief time, suddenly stopping and emptying your mind. Command yourself to "Stop!" right in the middle of one of your negative thoughts. By interrupting it you will gain an opportunity to replace it with another, more positive thought. Negative, unpleasant, enervating thoughts lead to negative, unpleasant, enervating emotions—which, in turn, deplete your body's natural tendency and energy to heal itself.

Positive, pleasant, and energetic thoughts do just the opposite. What are some of the replacement thoughts? Here is a listing of some useful ones:

"I'm going to be all right."
"I can beat this disease."
"This disease is not going to rule my life."
"I am cheerful and outgoing."
"I organize my life so that I am in control."
"I make plans to spend time with people I love."
"I try to stretch my mind every day to a new dimension."
"I am compassionate and caring for people who have problems."
"I am warm and witty and people enjoy being with me."
"I am resourceful and self-sufficient, and people look to me for advice."
"I am curious about the world around me."
"I am open and honest about my likes and dislikes."
"I have a solid plan for my life."

Help yourself.

CHAPTER 9

The Sex Connection

I have often wondered what might happen if some researchers proved, once and for all, without reservation, that sexual intercourse was the primary cause of bacterial cystitis. Would there suddenly be a sexual revolution with abstinence as the prevailing belief? I doubt it. Besides, it is quite clear that even a thorough pelvic exam can thrust bacteria into the bladder and touch off a full-blown infection for a cystitis-prone woman. Fortunately, sex is here to stay.

FREQUENT URINATION

Of greatest importance to the cystitis-prone woman are the times directly before and after intercourse. It is what you do—and what you *don't* do—that can decide whether you will be fit for another night of lovemaking or a trip to the doctor's office.

If for nothing else, pure comfort would suggest that you empty your bladder before intercourse. Certainly nothing is more distracting than the pressure of a full bladder at the height of arousal. But there *is* another reason: Voiding will flush out any bacteria that are lingering in the urethra, waiting to be transported into your bladder to begin multiplying even while you are making love. Then drink a glass of water so that before you nod off to sleep you can empty your bladder again. Frequent flushing is a key to avoiding cystitis. In most women, this process just eliminates the bacteria. Even if you are one of the segment of the female population with a highly receptive bladder, frequent urination will eliminate the urine that bacteria feed on as they multiply.

YOUR DIAPHRAGM

While we're in the preliminary stages, let's consider your contraceptives. Almost every form of birth control presents some unique problem: Oral contraceptives cause hormonal side effects in some women, nausea, breast tenderness, or mood changes. Others cannot use oral contraceptives because of age, medical history, or other reasons. Therefore, many women prefer barrier contraceptives, such as the diaphragm (see illustration page 83). But the trusty diaphragm causes problems, too. It is probably one of the major culprits in recurrent urinary tract infections. Pressing against the neck of the bladder, the diaphragm affects the bladder's normally efficient voiding process. The rate of urinary flow is decreased, pressure within the bladder is increased, and there is a high rate of urinary retention. Thus residual urine acts as a pool in which bacteria can grow. Also, increased turbulence in urine trying to get through a partly obstructed urethra may result in backflow, moving bacteria toward the bladder rather than out of the body.

Most physicians have been trained to fit a woman with the largest possible diaphragm. If recurrent cystitis results, however, a smaller diaphragm may have to be fitted. For prevention of pregnancy, the size really doesn't matter as much as the correct placement of the diaphragm, so that it covers—and holds—a spermicidal cream or jelly against the

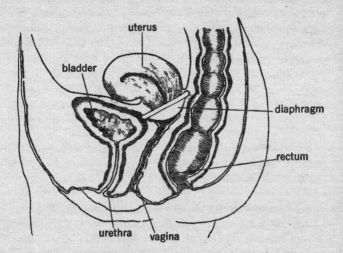

DIAPHRAGM PLACEMENT

cervix. A smaller-size diaphragm may reduce your chances of bacterial cystitis caused by urine retention in the bladder; it might also reduce the likelihood of cystitis brought out by a too-large diaphragm pressing against your urethra.

MAXIMIZE PLEASURE, MINIMIZE RISK

Whoever said that "position is everything in life" might well have been a woman with recurrent cystitis. Some positions in sexual intercourse cause more urethral irritation than others. Dagmar O'Connor, director of the sexual therapy program at St. Luke's Roosevelt Hospital in New York City, says that in her workshops one out of every seven women complains of cystitis. It may not always be bacterial cystitis, she says, but nonetheless, it is recurring irritation and much of it seems to stem from foreplay and intercourse. O'Connor suggests that lack of lubrication in many women may lead to irritation from a finger or penis rubbing away at dry surfaces. Nor does this only occur in "honeymoon" sexual encounters, with intercourse happening many times in a day, but even after a single time if the back-and-forth movement of finger or penis is difficult.

If a woman with a history of cystitis feels pressure on the bladder during intercourse, she should try to change her position until she feels comfortable.

Lucy, one young bride, quickly set about finding alternatives to the positions in intercourse that brought about problems. "Just changing the angle a little bit—from 90 degrees to something like 60 degrees—made all the difference," she says. Another position that was almost "risk free" put Lucy on top of her husband, Joe, giving her control of the depth of penetration. On some occasions they try a side-by-side position, a more relaxing type of intercourse, anyway, and one that reduces the incidence of irritation. "We're still experimenting," reports Lucy, happily.

We're talking here about the traditional reproductive mode of having sex—what O'Connor calls "the real thing." What about other forms of sexual experience such as anal sex, oral sex, and masturbation?

Sorry to say that they can still as easily lead to cystitis. Hands, lips, tongue, and vibrators can all transport microorganisms to the urethral opening. Some heterosexual couples practice anal intercourse. For the cystitis patient, this is not a good idea because it introduces high concentrations of *E. coli* bacteria to the external genital area. (Also there is a growing body of evidence connecting anal intercourse with AIDS transmission.)

A final word: Any sexual activity that irritates your urethra or bladder is bound, eventually, to irritate your relationship. Esther was one young woman who learned this hard lesson.

For several years, Esther had been victim of recurring cystitis attacks. Up until that time, she and her husband, Stan, had enjoyed a regular and satisfying sex life. But with the constantly returning infections, sex became a real turn-off for Esther, to the point where it was actually too painful physically as well as mentally. "The last doctor I saw suggested that I 'give it up for a while,' " Esther said. "But I had already stopped having intercourse, so that was no solution." The tensions and frustrations began to erupt in other areas of their marriage—fights about money, arguments about the children's grades in school, animosities about real and perceived inconsiderations. By the time Esther came to my office, the marriage was at the breaking point; in fact, Esther had moved into her family's home in a nearby suburb so that she could, as she put it, "sort it all out."

For Esther and Stan, the road back to a solid marital relationship was a difficult one. Both had been raised in an old-world type of home where sex was simply not a topic of conversation. Added to the poor communication between the two were certain uncertainties about basic anatomy and some ignorance about the disease that ostensibly was wrecking their marriage. But both were determined to save the union and consulted a sex therapist for help.

The counseling took several years to complete because

as it progressed Esther and Stan realized that Esther's cystitis had become the focal point for other, more subtle divisions. Esther hasn't had a cystitis attack in over a year. Better still, she and Stan recently celebrated their twentieth wedding anniversary with a ceremony to repeat their marriage vows.

I'm not suggesting that a program to prevent cystitis will magically solve all the problems in your marriage. But at least being free from pain and discomfort, from anxiety and tension, from confusion and doubt about the particular disease will leave you free to deal with the exigencies of your marriage or love union.

CHAPTER 10

The Diet Connection

There is much controversy today concerning the relationship between diet and/or nutritional status and urinary tract infection. Here are just a few snippets of advice picked up by my patients from magazine articles, books, and well-meaning friends and relatives: aim for an acid urine, aim for an alkaline urine, drink plenty of fluids, drink only water, load up with vitamins, load up with vitamin C, don't take any vitamin supplements. What is a woman to think?

Let me assure you right here that nothing you eat or drink is going to *cause* your infection. Foods and drinks can make you more susceptible to infection, however, or even increase the severity of the symptoms once infection has set in. What's more, some foods and beverages can, in some women, trigger cystitis symptoms without an actual infection simply because the waste products manufactured are highly irritating to the bladder. In some cases a real allergy to a food or beverage may be identified; it is unusual, however, for symptoms to appear *only* in the genitourinary tract and not as hives or respiratory distress, as well.

TRACKING DOWN THE CULPRITS

I wish that the food/sensitive bladder link could be clearly defined and that I could list for you 20 foods to avoid and that would be the end of it. But the old expression suggesting that one person's meat is another's poison could not be more fitting than in regard to cystitis symptoms.

One example that comes immediately to mind is orange juice. One of my patients, Melissa, discovered that every time she drank orange juice made from frozen concentrate she developed severe burning in her bladder. Fresh-squeezed orange juice, however, caused no more problem than tap water. For Dale, orange juice was only a problem when she took it first thing in the morning; at other times during the day she could drink it with no reaction.

FOOD/BEVERAGE SYMPTOM CHART

Food/Beverage	Quantity	Immediate Response	Delayed Response
Orange juice			
Other citrus			
Coffee			
Tea			
Cola drinks			
Diet cola drinks			
Food/beverages containing saccharine aspartame			
Alcohol			
Black pepper			
Hot peppers			
Other spices			
Salsa			

The point is that a specific food or beverage may not always cause an identical reaction in every person every time it is eaten or drunk. There is no denying, however, that certain foods and beverages are common culprits. I have listed these in a chart form to make them easy to pinpoint as problems for *you*. And don't be surprised if the reaction is not immediate. Foods and beverages are metabolized slower or faster depending on what else you have had to eat or drink. Sometimes it can take 12 hours or more for wastes to reach the bladder. If you are going to keep this sort of a food/beverage diary, be thorough. Don't dismiss a potential trigger just because you had it many hours prior to the onset of symptoms or because it was taken only in minute quantities.

If you are in the habit of eating several of these foods at the same time, you may have to do some dietary manipulating for purposes of identification. When I suggested this type of diary to Alyce, a patient who suffered from two or three attacks of cystitis-like symptoms each month, she was dismayed. "My favorite breakfast," she confessed, "is orange juice, cold cereal with strawberries, toast with strawberry jam, and coffee." For several days, Alyce eliminated all of the potentially offending items from her breakfast menu, then she started adding them back, one at a time. In Alyce's case, only the orange juice consistently produced symptoms. The patience it took to complete the trail was well worth it, she said, because she would have otherwise arbitrarily cut out all of her favorite breakfast treats.

EATING WISELY AND WELL

Dietary considerations for a cystitis-prone woman involve more than just eliminating certain problem foods from a diet. There is also a very positive aspect to diet that has to do with long-term nutritional status.

Frequently women who embark on a cystitis prevention program become keenly interested in their diets. Selecting meals and menus, does, after all, give a firm sense of control, and people like to have that. Very often I refer my patients to Lynne M. Perkins (R.D., M.S., M.A.), a registered dietitian who is a consulting nutritionist in private practice in New York City. Diets based on unproven theories are anathema to Perkins, who believes that people sometimes become fixated on such fad and gimmick diets, and thereby tend to turn the uncomplicated practice of eating well into a complicated and even harmful procedure.

Perkins's sensible approach to diet and nutrition has helped a great many women not only gain control over their cystitis symptoms but also their overall nutritional status. Here are some of her suggestions for cystitis-prone women:

Drink Plenty of Water

Six to eight glasses a day is the absolute minimum as an effective preventive measure for holding cystitis in abeyance. If infection sets in, the amount must be increased to 10 glasses a day at very least. If you work in an office, keep a container of water at your desk so that you can sip throughout the day. If your work involves traveling, keep a Thermos of cool water with you wherever you go. Be sure your water intake is evenly spaced throughout the day; drinking a large glass all at once will leave you feeling bloated and uncomfortable, and you'll be less likely to continue the routine. Chances are you will feel slightly full anyway for the first few days that you increase your water intake, but this feeling will disappear as soon as your body adapts to the increase in fluid.

Contrary to what most people think, Perkins says, you *can* drink too much water, although it is unlikely that you will. For the most part, your body will simply get rid of any water that it does not need through exhalation, perspiration, and, more important, excretion. For the average woman, more than 10 to 12 glasses of water a day could produce some negative side effects. An exception might be a woman who perspires a great deal because of strenuous physical activity. With an adequate water intake, the natural process of urination will flush out the harmful bacteria that have found a way into your bladder. Drinking too little water is a more common problem. Some women actually may go weeks at a time without drinking a glass of water, assuming that other beverages will suffice to keep them hydrated. Coffee, tea, and colas are not a substitute for water. In fact, these beverages may increase the body's need for water.

Too little water results in a very concentrated urine in which bacteria will quickly multiply. Initially, while you are still conscious of an increased intake of water, it might help to break the monotony by switching to bottled mineral water every so often. Soon, though, you will forget all about it and sipping at plain tap water will be a natural part of your routine.

Monitor Intake of Acidic Foods and Beverages

Logic might suggest that eating oranges, grapefruit, and other acidic foods will irritate your bladder. This is generally not true, or at least not across the board for all acidic foods and all women. If you are faithful about your food diary, you will soon discover which foods trigger symptoms for you. If foods don't cause a problem, by all means leave them in your diet; otherwise you might be unnecessarily eliminating an important source of nutrients.

Drink Cranberry Juice

For years, conventional wisdom about warding off cystitis or arresting it in its tracks advised drinking large amounts of cranberry juice. Until recently, the effectiveness of cranberry juice was explained by its power to render urine highly acidic and, therefore, quite inhospitable to bacteria. What never made sense was that plenty of other juices had the same acidic effect on urine, yet no other juice was capable of keeping bacteria at bay. Recently, it has been found (in female mice, anyway) that cranberry juice actually diminishes the ability of bacteria to adhere to the lining of the bladder. When the bacteria are unable to latch onto the bladder lining, it is easier for the water, which the cystitis-prone woman is now taking in large quantities throughout the day, to wash the bacteria away. In effect, then, the cranberry juice changes a cystitis-prone bladder to a more normal state.

Eliminate Coffee, Tea, and Cola Drinks

Many women assume that as long as they are taking in liquids, it makes no difference what the liquids are. Such an assumption can lead to plenty of trouble, bladder-wise. Coffee, tea, and colas contain caffeine, which is a strong stimulant. Although the added stimulus on the bladder is, in theory, good in that it will increase frequency of urination and thus give bacteria little chance to multiply, it doesn't work that way unless large quantities of water are being taken in at the same time. These beverages also contain tannic acid which can be highly irritating to a sensitive bladder. Better leave these beverages to others and concentrate on water and cranberry juice.

Try Vitamin C Supplements

Some women swear by a daily supplement of vitamin C, whereas others see no change at all. If you have found that a daily vitamin C supplement is helpful in managing cystitis, continue with your routine. Check with your doctor if you plan on taking more than 500 milligrams a day, however. For many women, large amounts of vitamin C cause adverse reactions such as diarrhea and—pay attention here— urinary tract irritation or kidney stones.

Limit Other Vitamin and Mineral Supplements

There are numerous theories at large today about the positive effect of megadoses of vitamins and minerals on the immune system. It is a long leap of faith between theory and proven fact, and it is probably safer to moderate your dosages of vitamin and mineral supplements. And don't forget to take them with food and plenty of water to make sure that they are metabolized properly. High doses of water-soluble B vitamins taken without an adequate amount of water can be an irritant to your bladder. Perkins's advice: Be moderate and drink plenty of water with such vitamins and after.

Learn to Like Yogurt

Although yogurt is not directly connected to management of cystitis, it is of great value in the event that you find yourself on a course of antibiotics. The problem with such drugs is that while they are eliminating bacteria from your bladder, they are also changing the bacterial flora in the large intestine and bowel. Four to eight ounces of yogurt (plain is best) will help to replace these good bacteria. Many doctors also recommend douching with yogurt to reduce the possibility of vaginal infection, which may be an adverse effect of antibiotics taken to get rid of bladder infection.

Stay Well-Nourished

Although super doses of vitamins and mineral supplements will probably not enhance your immune system, an inadequate nutritional status will leave you more susceptible to infection. To stay well-nourished, include in your diet plenty of whole grains, vegetables, legumes, fruits and foods to provide protein such as meat, fish, eggs, dairy products, and tofu. If your diet includes a fair amount of alcoholic beverages, you are likely to be missing valuable nutrients as well as increasing your body's need for such nutrients.

It is beyond the scope of this book to go into dietary plans, menus, and recipes. However, if you feel that you could use advice in this area, contact the American Dietetic Association, 430 North Michigan Avenue, Chicago, IL 60601. They will send you a list of consulting nutritionists in private practice in your area. Look for those who are registered dieticians (R.D.), as well as having graduate training in clinical nutrition (M.S. or Ph.D.)

A Guide to Common Prescription Drugs

In treating a woman with cystitis, a doctor has three goals: one, to eradicate the bacteria in the bladder that are causing the infection; two, to try to avoid disruption of useful bacteria elsewhere in the body; and, three, to prescribe a course of treatment that will be within the patient's financial means.

Taking these factors into account, the range of antibacterial drugs is narrowed. Here are the drugs that I use most often in treating bacterial cystitis.

NITROFURANTOIN

What are the common names for nitrofurantoin?
Furadantin, Macrodantin

What should I tell my doctor before he or she prescribes nitrofurantoin?
Tell your doctor if you have kidney disease, if you are allergic to this agent, or if you are pregnant and near term. Nitrofurantoin should not be taken if any of these conditions exist.

In what forms is nitrofurantoin available?
Nitrofurantoin comes in capsules, tablets, or oral suspension.

The usual dosage is:

Adult: 50 to 100 mg. 4 times per day

Child (over age 3 months): 2 to 3 mg. per pound of body weight in 4 divided doses

Child (under age 3 months): Not recommended

Nitrofurantoin may be used in lower doses over a long period by people with chronic urinary infections.

How should I take nitrofurantoin?

Nitrofurantoin may be taken with food or milk to help decrease stomach upset, loss of appetite, nausea, or other gastrointestinal symptoms. Be sure to continue taking this medicine at least 3 days after you stop experiencing symptoms of urinary tract infection.

Does Nitrofurantoin have any side effects?

The possible side effects of this drug include loss of appetite, nausea, vomiting, stomach pain, and diarrhea. Some people develop hepatitislike symptoms. Side effects are generally less prominent when Macrodantin (large crystal form of nitrofurantoin) is used rather than Furadantin (regular crystal size).

Be sure to inform your doctor immediately if you experience any of the following while using nitrofurantoin: fever, chills, cough, chest pain, difficulty in breathing. If these occur in the first week of therapy, they can generally be resolved by stopping the medication. If they occur after a longer time, they can be more serious because they develop more slowly and are more difficult to associate with the drug. Other adverse effects can include: rashes, itching, asthmatic attacks in patients with a history of asthma, drug fever, symptoms similar to arthritis, jaundice (yellowing of the whites of the eyes and/or skin), headache, dizziness, drowsiness, temporary loss of hair. The oral liquid form of nitrofurantoin can stain your teeth if you don't swallow the medicine rapidly. Nitrofurantoin may also give your urine a brownish color, but this is not dangerous.

How closely should I keep in touch with my doctor while I'm taking nitrofurantoin?
If your symptoms show no sign of improvement after a few days of treatment, or you experience any adverse side effects, consult your physician.

Should I restrict any foods or drinks while I'm taking nitro-furantoin?
There are no restrictions.

SULFISOXAZOLE

What are the common brand names for sulfisoxazole?
Azo Gantrisin (also contains phenazopyridine hydrochloride, a urinary analgesic), Gantrisin

What should I tell my doctor before he or she prescribes sulfisoxazole?
Be sure to tell your doctor about any asthma or allergic reactions you've experienced, especially to sulfonamides, furosemide, thiazide diuretics, dapsone, sulfoxone, oral antidiabetics, or glaucoma medication such as acetazolamide, dichlorphenamide, methazolamide, or ethoxzolamide. If you have had kidney disease, liver disease, intestinal or urinary tract obstruction, hay fever, strep throat, porphyria, anemia produced by any drug, or G6PD deficiency, your doctor must be told. Also, inform your doctor if you are, or even think you are pregnant, if you plan to become pregnant, or if you are breast-feeding a baby.

Tell your doctor about all prescription and nonprescription medications you are currently taking, especially any of the following: paraaminobenzoic acid (PABA); isoniazid;

diuretics; digoxin; oxyphenbutazone; penicillins; phenyl-butazone; methenamine; methotrexate; phenytoin; proben-ecid; sulfinpyrazone; barbiturates; oral anticoagulants; oral hypoglycemics; aspirin or other salicylates; or medication to make your urine more alkaline such as sodium citrate, potassium citrate, citric acid, or sodium bicarbonate. Ask your doctor or pharmacist to identify your medication if you are not sure what kind you take.

If you are allergic to sulfonamides, you should not take this drug. If you are late in pregnancy, if you are breast-feeding an infant, or if you've had porphyria or intestinal or urinary tract obstruction, you should not take this drug. Infants under one month of age should not be given this drug. When taking sulfisoxazole, avoid taking large doses of vitamin C.

In what forms is sulfisoxazole available?
Sulfisoxazole is available in tablets, pediatric suspension, and syrup.
The usual dosage is:
Adult: first dose, 4 to 8 tablets; then 2 to 3 tablets 4 times per day (not to exceed 12 tablets daily)
Child (over 50 pounds): Liquid suspension, 1 teaspoon 4 times per day; liquid syrup, 2 teaspoons 4 times per day.

How should I take sulfisoxazole?
Take this drug with a full, 8-ounce glass of water on an empty stomach, 1 or 2 hours before meals. Try not to miss any doses. Drink at least 8 full glasses of water or other liquids each day. If you are taking the liquid form of Gantrisin, shake the bottle well and measure the liquid in a specially marked spoon or dropper; an ordinary teaspoon may not be accurate.

If you miss a dose, take the missed dose as soon as possi-ble, unless it is close to the time for your next dose. In that case, if you are taking two doses a day, space the missed dose and the next dose 4 to 6 hours apart; if you're taking three or more doses a day, space the missed dose and the next dose 2 to 4 hours apart, or double the next dose. Then return to your regular dosing schedule.

Does sulfisoxazole have any side effects?
This drug can cause loss of appetite, nausea, vomiting, diarrhea, difficult urination, dizziness, headache, depression, insomnia, and a brown discoloration of the urine. The discoloration is harmless. As your body adjusts to this drug, these side effects should disappear. If you feel dizzy, sit or lie down for a while, get up slowly, and be careful on stairs.

It is especially important that you report to your doctor any of the following: hallucinations; hives; itching or rash; increased sensitivity to sunlight; severe reaction to the sun; an unexplained sore throat or fever; mouth sores; unusual bleeding or bruising; unusual fatigue or weakness; yellowing of the eyes or the skin; aching muscles and joints; swallowing or breathing difficulties; paleness, redness, blistering, or loosening of the skin; blood in the urine; swelling of the face; swelling in the front part of the neck; lower back pain; a painful burning sensation during urination; tingling in the hands or feet; hearing loss; loss of coordination; ringing in the ears; or hair loss.

How closely should I keep in touch with my doctor while I'm taking sulfisoxazole?
Contact your doctor if your symptoms get worse or show no improvement. If you are taking sulfisoxazole for a prolonged period, your doctor will probably want to see you regularly to monitor your progress and to conduct blood cell counts and liver and kidney function tests.

Should I restrict any foods or drinks while I'm taking sulfisoxazole?
There are no food restrictions. Consult your doctor before you

drink any alcoholic beverages while you are taking this drug.

AMOXICILLIN

Under what brand names is amoxicillin available?
Amoxil, Polymox, Trimox, Wymox

What should I tell my doctor before he or she prescribes amoxicillin?
It is very important that you tell your doctor about any asthma or allergic reactions you've experienced, especially those caused by other antibiotics, penicillin, or cephalosporins. If you are allergic to these, you may be allergic to amoxicillin. Also, let your doctor know if you've ever had eczema, hives, skin rashes, or kidney or liver disease. Finally, tell your doctor about all prescription and nonprescription medications you are taking, especially penicillin, tetracycline, sulfa drugs, chloramphenicol, probenecid, or erythromycin. The effect of ampicillin can be significantly reduced when taken with other antibiotics.

In what forms is amoxicillin available?
Amoxicillin comes in: capsules (various colors) of 250 mg. or 500 mg.; oral suspension, 125 mg. per teaspoonful or 250 mg. per teaspoonful; and pediatric drops, 50 mg. per ml. The typical dosage is:
Adult: 250 to 500 mg. 3 to 4 times a day
Child (44 pounds and over): 250 to 500 mg. every 6 hours
Child (under 44 pounds): 50 to 100 mg. every 6 to 8 hours
Amoxicillin should be stored at room temperature.

How should I take amoxicillin?
Amoxicillin should be taken at evenly spaced intervals around the clock as directed by your doctor. It can be taken on a full or empty stomach. If you are taking amoxicillin in sus-

pension form, shake the bottle well and measure the liquid with a marked spoon; an ordinary teaspoon may not be accurate. If you are giving the pediatric solution to a child, measure it in a dropper and place it directly on the child's tongue. If necessary, the solution can be mixed with milk, juice, water, or soft drinks, but make sure the full dose is swallowed. If you forget to take your prescribed dose, take the missed dose immediately. If you did not remember to take the missed dose until it was almost time for your next dose, however, space that next dose about halfway through the regular interval between doses. Then return to your regular schedule. Do not skip a dose or the effect of the antibiotic will be severely reduced.

Does Amoxicillin have any side effects?
Amoxicillin can cause diarrhea and nausea. As your body adjusts to this drug, these side effects should disappear. To reduce stomach upset, take amoxicillin with food unless your doctor orders otherwise.

Be sure to tell your doctor about any severe or persistent side effects. It's especially important to report to your doctor any of the following irregular reactions to the drug: a dark-colored tongue; yellow-green stools; vaginal discharge; hives, itching, or skin rash; congestion in the lungs; sore throat; fever; difficult breathing; abdominal pain; severe or persistent diarrhea; vomiting; joint pain; difficult swallowing; wheezing; swelling of the face; swelling of the joints or lymph glands; weakness, dizziness, or fainting; rectal or vaginal itching; or sores in the mouth.

How closely should I keep in touch with my doctor while I'm taking amoxicillin?
If there is no improvement in your symptoms or if they grow worse, then you should contact your doctor. If you are treated with amoxicillin for a prolonged period, your doctor may want you to undergo regular tests for liver and kidney function.

Should I restrict any foods or drinks?
There are no food or drink restrictions.

PENICILLIN VK

What are the common brand names for penicillin VK?
Betapen-VK, Pen-Vee K, SK-Penicillin VK, V-Cillin K, Veetids

What should I tell my doctor before he or she prescribes penicillin VK?
Be sure to tell your doctor about any asthma or allergic reactions you've experienced, especially to other forms of penicillin, neomycin, and antibiotics of the cephalosporin family. You should not take penicillin VK if you have ever had an allergic reaction to this drug or to any other form of penicillin or penicillamine. Also, let your doctor know if you have had any liver or kidney disease or any disorder that involves vomiting or diarrhea. Also, tell your doctor about any prescription or nonprescription drugs you are taking, especially any of the following: antibiotics, especially oral neomycin, erythromycin, chloramphenicol, and tetracycline; sulfa drugs; gout medications such as probenecid; aspirin; phenylbutazone; indomethacin; or sulfinpyrazone. Ask your doctor or pharmacist to identify your medication if you are not sure what kind you take.

In what forms is penicillin VK available?
Penicillin VK comes in: tablets (various colors) of 125 mg., 250 mg., and 500 mg.; oral solution, 125 mg. per teaspoonful, or 250 mg. per teaspoonful. The usual dosage is 125 to 250 mg. every 6 to 8 hours for 10 days. Oral solution penicillin VK may have to be stored in a refrigerator. The bottle should be labeled to that effect and the information should be available on the prescription label.

How should I take penicillin VK?
This drug should be taken at evenly spaced intervals around the clock as prescribed by your physician. Penicillin VK is usually taken with a full glass of water on an empty stomach 1 hour before or 2 hours after a meal. If the drug upsets your stomach, ask your doctor if you can take the medication with food. If you are taking the liquid form of this drug, shake it well and measure it with a specially marked spoon or dropper. Take all doses of this medication on schedule.

If you miss a dose, take the missed dose immediately. If you did not remember to take the missed dose until it was almost time for your next dose, however, space that next dose about halfway through the regular interval between doses. Then return to your regular dosing schedule. Do not skip a dose.

Does penicillin VK have any side effects?
Until your body adjusts to the drug, penicillin VK can cause upset stomach, nausea, vomiting, and diarrhea. If the medication upsets your stomach, ask your doctor if you can take the drug with food.

Be sure to tell your doctor about any severe or persistent side effects from penicillin VK. It's especially important to report to your doctor any of the following: marked change in stools; vaginal discharge; discolored or darkened tongue; frequent vomiting; wheezing; skin rash; hives; itching; swelling of the face; difficult urination; fever; chills; sore throat; muscle aches; lung congestion; dizziness; weakness; bloating; joint pain; difficulty swallowing; abdominal pain; swelling of the joints or lymph glands; sore mouth or tongue; or loss of consciousness.

How closely should I keep in touch with my doctor while I'm taking penicillin VK?
If your symptoms show no sign of improvement after a few days of treatment, or if they seem to get worse, contact your

doctor. If you are taking this drug over a long period of time, your doctor may want to take blood cell counts and tests of liver and kidney function.

Should I restrict any foods or drinks while I'm taking penicillin VK?
There are no restrictions.

CEPHALEXIN
(and other cephalosporins)

Under what brand name is cephalexin available?
Keflex

What should I tell my doctor before he or she prescribes cephalexin (or other cephalosporins)?
Be sure to tell your doctor about any asthma, hay fever, or allergic reactions you have experienced, especially to cephalexin, to other antibiotics of the cephalosporin family, and to penicillin. Tell your doctor if you have ever had kidney disease or diabetes, and inform your doctor if you are, or even think you are, pregnant, or if you are breast-feeding a baby. Tell your doctor if you are using any prescription or nonprescription medications, especially other antibiotics such as gentamicin, colistin, and polyyxin B; diuretics; anticoagulants; or probenecid. Ask your doctor or pharmacist to identify your medication so that you will be sure what you are taking.

In what forms is cephalexin available?
Cephalexin comes in capsule (white and green), 250 mg.; double strength capsule (light green and dark green) contains 500 mg., and quadruple strength tablet (green, capsule strength), 1 g. It is also available in pediatric drops, 100

mg. per ml., and oral suspension, 125 mg. per teaspoonful
and 250 mg. per teaspoonful.

How should I take cephalexin?
You should take the capsule and tablet form of this medication (and other cephalosporins) with a full 8-ounce glass of
water. All forms of the medication may be taken on either a
full or empty stomach, but if the medication causes an upset
stomach, take it with food. If you are taking the liquid form
of the medication, use a marked spoon because an ordinary
teaspoon may not be accurate. Take the drug at evenly spaced
intervals around the clock as prescribed by your doctor. Try
to take all doses on time.

Does cephalexin have any side effects?
This drug (and other cephalosporins) can cause diarrhea,
nausea, vomiting, abdominal pain, fatigue, headache, heart-
burn, loss of appetite, anal and genital itching, and dizziness. These side effects should disappear as your body
adjusts to the drug. If you experience dizziness, lie down
for a while.

*How closely should I keep in touch with my doctor while I'm
taking cephalexin?*
If your symptoms get worse or show no improvement, you
should contact your doctor. Also, if you are taking the medication for a long period of time, your doctor will probably
want to give you periodic blood cell counts and liver and kidney function tests.

*Should I restrict any foods or drinks while I'm taking
cephalexin?*
There are no food restrictions with this drug (or other cephalosporins). Check with your doctor before drinking alcoholic beverages while taking cephalexin (or other cephalosporins).

SULFAMETHOXAZOLE PLUS TRIMETHOPRIM

What are the common brand names for sulfamethoxazole plus trimethoprim?
Bactrim, Septra, Septra DS, Cotrim, Cotrim D.S.

What should I tell my doctor before he or she prescribes sulfamethoxazole plus trimethoprim?
Be sure to tell you doctor about any asthma or allergic reactions you have experienced, especially to trimethoprim, sulfonamides, furosemide or thiazide diuretics, acetazolomide, dapsone, sulfoxone, oral antidiabetics, or oral glaucoma drugs. Tell your doctor if you have ever had kidney disease, liver disease, porphyria, folate deficiency, or anemia. Inform your doctor if you are, or even think you are, pregnant, or if you are breast-feeding a baby. Tell your doctor if you are using any prescription or nonprescription medications, especially anticoagulants, barbiturates, oral diabetes drugs, cyclophosphamide, diuretics, methotrexate, methenamine, penicillin, oxacillin, phenytoin, paraldehyde, isoniazid, probenecid, sulfinpyrazone, local anesthetics, medication to make your urine more alkaline such as sodium bicarbonate or sodium citrate, paraaminobenzoic acid (PABA), phenylbutazone, or oxyphenbutazone. Ask your doctor or pharmacist to identify your medication so that you will be sure what you are taking.

In what forms is sulfamethoxazole plus trimethoprim available?
Sulfamethoxazole plus trimethoprim comes in tablets 400 mg. of sulfamethoxazole and 80 mg. of trimethoprim. Double strength contains double the milligrams. Liquid contains 200 mg. of sulfamethoxazole and 40 mg. of trimethoprim per teaspoonful.

How should I take sulfamethoxazole plus trimethoprim?
You should take this medication with a full, 8-ounce glass of water. In addition, drink at least eight full glasses of water or other liquids each day. Take the drug at evenly spaced times around the clock; for example, "one tablet twice a day" means every 12 hours. If you are using the liquid form, shake well before pouring and measure the dose accurately. Be sure to continue taking the medication for the complete time your doctor prescribed it, even if you are feeling better and your symptoms have disappeared.

Does sulfamethoxazole plus trimethoprim have any side effects?
This drug can cause diarrhea, nausea, stomach pain, vomiting, vertigo, headache, dizziness, loss of appetite, and extra sensitivity to the sun. As your body adjusts to the drug, however, these side effects should disappear. To reduce stomach upset, take the drug with milk or food. If you experience dizziness, lie down for a while. To protect yourself from severe sunburn, limit your exposure to the sun and use an effective sunscreen, but not one that contains paraaminobenzoic acid (PABA).

How closely should I keep in touch with my doctor while I'm taking sulfamethoxazole plus trimethoprim?
If your symptoms get worse, or show no improvement, you should contact your doctor. Also, if you are taking the medication for a long period of time, your doctor will probably want to give you periodic blood cell counts and liver and kidney function tests.

Should I restrict any foods or drinks while I'm taking sulfamethoxazole plus trimethoprim?
There are no food restrictions. Check with your doctor before drinking alcoholic beverages while taking sulfamethoxazole plus trimethoprim.

There is one additional drug—not an antibiotic—that I frequently prescribe for the relief of pain during a cystitis attack.

PHENAZOPYRIDINE HYDROCHLORIDE

Under what brand names is phenazopyridine hydrochloride available?
Pyridium, Urogesic. (It is also combined with anitbacterial agents in Azo Gantanol, Azo-Gantrisin, Pyridium Plus, and Thiosulfil-A.)

What should I tell my doctor before he or she prescribes phenazopyridine hydrochloride?
Make sure you tell your doctor about any asthma or allergic reactions you've experienced, especially to phenazopyridine, and if you've had either hepatitis or kidney disease. If you are allergic to phenazopyridine, or if you suffer from severe kidney disease, you should not take this drug. Inform your doctor if you are, or even think you are, pregnant, or if you are breast-feeding a baby.

You must also tell your doctor about all prescription and nonprescription medications you are currently taking. Ask your doctor or pharmacist to identify your medication if you are not sure what kind you take.

In what forms is phenazopyridine hydrochloride available?
This drug comes in tablets of 100 or 200 mg. The usual dosage is: 200 mg. 3 times per day.

How should I take phenazopyridine hydrochloride?
Take it with a full glass of water either with your meal or directly after it. If you miss a dose, take the missed dose as

soon as possible, unless it is close to the time for your next dose. In that case, don't take the missed dose at all. Do not double the next dose, but go back to your regular dosing schedule.

Does this drug have any side effects?
Phenazopyridine hydrochloride can cause dizziness, headache, indigestion, stomach cramps, or stomach pain. As your body adjusts to this drug, however, these side effects should disappear. It may turn urine a harmless reddish-orange color and so may stain clothing. If you feel dizzy, sit or lie down for a while, get up slowly, and be careful on stairs. To reduce stomach upset, take this drug with food, unless your doctor orders otherwise.

If any of the side effects are severe or persistent, report them to your doctor immediately. It is especially important that you report to your doctor any unusually dark or bloody urine, excessive fatigue, yellowing of the eyes or skin, or rash.

How closely should I keep in touch with my doctor while I'm taking phenazopyridine hydrochloride?
If there is no improvement in your symptoms or if they become worse, you should contact your doctor. If you take phenazopyridine hydrochloride for a long time, your doctor may want to monitor your progress and do periodic blood cell count and liver function tests.

Should I restrict any foods or drinks while I'm taking phenazopyridine hydrochloride?
There are no food restrictions while taking phenazopyridine. Consult your doctor before you drink any alcoholic beverages while you are taking this drug.

CHAPTER 12

A Dose of Good Advice

If, in spite of your well-planned prevention program to avoid cystitis, it happens anyway, that could be bad news. The good news, however, is that the disease is extremely sensitive to drug therapy, especially if it is caught at the first sign of infection.

USE DRUGS EFFECTIVELY

Very often, a person can sabotage the potential effectiveness of a medicine, or even turn it into a dangerous foe. How? By taking medicine at the wrong time, in the wrong way, or with other substances that may be wrong in partnership with the particular medicine.

For example, orange juice or other acidic fruit and vegetable juices may help to get the antibiotic down easier, but it may diminish the effectiveness of the pill when it gets into your system. Dairy products bind to some medications, and make them less effective.

The obvious consequence of not taking medication properly is a delay in recovery, which, put another way, means prolonged suffering. Furthermore, some drugs can cause unpleasant side effects on their own. Much of the potential down side of strong medicine can be avoided if you make absolutely sure you know all you need to know about the drug.

The key to how well a drug works is a process called bioavailability. Simply stated, this means the percentage of a drug contained in a product that enters the system in an active form. Interestingly, this is not the same in all people and the amount is influenced by a number of factors. For example, a woman who weighs 100 pounds will probably experience faster and better results from an antibiotic than another woman who weighs 180 pounds, assuming the dosage is exactly the same. This is because the heavier woman has a slower metabolism, which means that drugs (and food, too) are broken down more slowly in the system for use. But what if the thinner woman smokes? And what if she is in the habit of having several cocktails every night? And what if she is taking another prescription or over-the-counter drug? All of these factors can affect the amount of the medication that gets into the bloodstream.

DO YOU COMMUNICATE WITH YOUR DOCTOR?

Are you a runner? Do you skip meals frequently? Is caffeine a mainstay of your day? It is crucial that your doctor know all of these things. Don't consider anything too insignificant to mention while you are in your doctor's office, talking about the prescription he or she is writing out.

Communication (or rather the lack of it) is probably the main reason why many drug regimens fail. This breakdown in dialogue between you and your doctor can be traced, more often than not, to the combination of circumstances that occurs when you are in his or her office. You are in pain and you are preoccupied with your condition. At the same time, your doctor wants to get you started on your medication as quickly as possible. The result is a great void in understanding and an even greater chance for what is known in the medical profession as "untoward effects."

The best way to avoid crossed signals is to prepare yourself before your office visit with a list of questions. Earlier in this book, you began to understand the importance of listing your exact symptoms in order to assist your doctor in diagnosis. Now I suggest a list of questions that you should ask your doctor if it becomes evident that you will need an anti-infective to halt the progression of your infection.

What is the purpose of this medication?
Ask your doctor to explain why you have developed this infection and why you need this particular drug to combat it. Do not accept "It will make you feel better," as an explanation. Be certain, too, that you know the exact brand name of the medication you are going to be taking (or the generic name if that is what you will be taking).

What should I do about side effects?
In the previous chapter, I summarized the most common effects and side effects of the drugs usually prescribed for bacterial cystitis. Some women react to antibiotics with loss of appetite or nausea, and how this is overcome depends entirely on the person. Sometimes food helps and sometimes it makes the problem worse; be assured that the gastrointestinal upset is temporary. What antibiotics do affect is the bacterial balance in other parts of your body, perhaps leaving you vulnerable to infections elsewhere. This is especially true in the vagina; a regimen of antibiotics to halt a cystitis attack may leave you open to vaginitis. Yogurt often helps to maintain bacterial "flora" (this useful food was discussed in Chapter 10). Your doctor may tell you that side effects will be transient, but pin that statement down. After all, it is

important to know at what point you should realistically be concerned that the drug is working against you. Be sure you and your doctor discuss any allergic reactions you have had to other drugs—any other drugs, not only antibiotics. There are many drugs available to treat cystitis; the point is to find the best one for you.

How will I know if the medicine is working?
Sometimes you will feel better right away as the antibiotic begins to fight the infection in your system. But what you may not know is that the drug is continuing to work, even though you are not aware of it. Many people stop taking their medicine as soon as they feel well, even though they still have several days' worth of pills left. Your doctor has decided on a certain length of time for you to remain on this medicine given your present condition and past history. Use up the entire prescribed dose. They won't do you any good in the container on the shelf, anyway.

When and how should I take this medicine?
I have briefly suggested all the factors that come to play upon the effectiveness of your medication. Your doctor must outline your routine for you so that you understand it totally. Should your medicine be taken on an empty stomach or with food? What about a four-time-a-day prescription; does this mean once every 6 hours or four times during your waking hours? Make sure you understand it all before you head for the pharmacy to fill the prescription.

Will this drug interact with other drugs, food, or alcohol?
There isn't a single drug that doesn't interact in some fashion, so get it straight right up front as to what this medicine will clash with. The one thing I would advise against no matter what antiinfective you end up with is alcohol. Alcohol makes a bad mixer with so many medicines that it is common sense to abstain during the course of your drug regimen.

Will this medicine interfere with other laboratory tests?
If for some reason you will be undergoing tests for another
medical condition, your doctor must know this so that the
drug can be adjusted accordingly, or so that the test results
can be interpreted in light of your medical regimen.

How shall I store this drug?
Keep all medicines away from the reach of small children.
Some drugs do better kept in the refrigerator, some are best
stored at room temperature. Ask your physician or pharmacist about storing the drug you have received.

*Can I share this medication with someone who has the same
disease?*
Temptation is great to lend a couple of pills when someone
you know develops symptoms similar to yours. Don't do it.
Your symptoms may be the same, but the illness may be
different. What's more, your reactions to a drug may be totally unalike, and a safe drug for one person may set off an
allergic reaction in another.

Is there a generic form of this drug available?
Most drugs (except the very newest ones on the market)
are available in generic form. On the plus side, the cost may
be substantially lower than with a brand name drug. On the
other hand, studies have shown that in some instances,
generic drugs are *not* exact equivalents medically, opening
up questions as to how it will work for you. Also when I write
one prescription in generic form, I advise my patients that
the pharmacist may not pass along the savings to you—so
check with your pharmacist.

PART III

Cystitis Under Special Circumstances

CHAPTER 13

With Child, Without Cystitis

A woman who has recently learned that she is pregnant is preoccupied with thoughts of names for a baby, nursery furnishings, infant nutrition, and parenting techniques. Certainly the last thing most women consider is cystitis, which is unfortunate because statistics show that between 2 and 10 percent of all pregnant woman develop bacteriuria, which means that they are carrying bacteria somewhere in the urinary tract. Most of these pregnant women are asymptomatic; they do not suffer from the typical pains and distresses that plague a victim of bacterial cystitis. But the infection is there, nonetheless. And so are the dangers.

Cystitis during pregnancy may lead to premature labor and premature delivery if not treated promptly. Asymptomatic infection, therefore, is a serious problem in pregnancy, one that women should take steps to avoid or stop in its tracks if it does occur.

Gayle B. is one of the lucky women who avoided the potential complications of cystitis in pregnancy. When I first saw Gayle as a patient she had already suffered through nearly eight years of fairly regular episodes of cystitis. She was 24 at the time and eagerly opted for the prevention program that I proposed. The next time I saw

Gayle was a year later when I confirmed that she was pregnant. She informed me that the prevention program had been totally successful and that she felt that she might never have to face another bladder infection. Certainly she looked to be in robust health during that particular visit. Her energy level was high, her skin clear and glowing, and, as she put it, "I don't have a complaint in the world." Her general physical examination seemed to bear out that assessment. But when the urinalysis report came back, I saw that there was considerable cause for concern: Gayle's urine sample was full of bacteria. At first she couldn't believe the diagnosis. "If anyone knows the discomfort of cystitis, I do," she said. "I have not had a single feeling of urgency or burning or pain for two years. And I would have surely recognized the symptoms during the past months, when I have been so keenly aware of everything that is happening in my body."

But that is part of the deceptive nature of cystitis in pregnancy—it often appears without a single warning sign. In pregnant women who have a history of cystitis, urine samples should be taken at each visit, even from those who appear to be in robust health. No one is absolutely sure just why bacteriuria is so prevalent in pregnancy. For a long while, the theory was that the growing fetus exerted pressure on the bladder, causing urinary retention and growth of bacteria. Then researchers began to notice that infection sometimes occurs even before the fetus is large enough to press against anything. At the moment, both theories are supported in the medical community. Furthermore, a pregnant woman's immune system undergoes many changes and she is, in many cases, more susceptible to infection.

In a nonpregnant woman, the diagnosis of bacteria in the urine—with or without symptoms—calls for a course of treatment with an antimicrobial or antiinfective agent. As I have pointed out in previous chapters, several drugs have been proved to be effective in eradicating bacteria, and the choice depends on the patient's state of health, desired potency of drug, and cost. With a pregnant woman, the considerations are not so simple. The most common therapies in the treatment of pregnant women with cystitis are ampicillin or amoxicillin, forms of penicillin, and cephalosporins.

The facts surrounding bacteriuria in pregnant women are promising in one respect: If it is detected early enough and treated, no harm will come to either the fetus or the mother. Following are some of the questions commonly asked by pregnant women concerning cystitis. I think the answers will be helpful to you.

Question: I have a history of cystitis. Do I need to take special precautions now that I am pregnant?
I suggest frequent urine cultures for a pregnant woman with a history of cystitis even if there are no symptoms. Of course, if you develop any symptoms of cystitis during pregnancy, see your doctor as soon as you possibly can so that a urine culture may be done and treatment begun promptly if results are positive.

Question: How often do I need to visit my doctor.
Usually every two to four weeks until the last two months of pregnancy, when visits should be spaced every one or two weeks. Again if you are not feeling well or experience any symptoms that suggest you are having an episode of cystitis, call your doctor immediately.

Question: I seem to be retaining water now that I am pregnant. Am I more in danger of developing bladder infection?
No, but it is important to continue drinking at least 8 glasses of water a day even if you feel you are retaining water.

Question: I am drinking a lot of milk because I think that my baby needs the calcium. Is this a good thing?

You are quite right, your baby will benefit from your increased intake of milk and milk products. But remember, milk is not a substitute for water, so be sure you meet your daily quota of water in your plan to avoid cystitis.

Question: What if the cystitis is cured early in my pregnancy and then recurs close to my delivery date?
There is no avoiding it: You will have to be treated with antibiotics again. All the more reason to be very careful and to follow a prevention plan.

Question: Can my baby catch cystitis from me?
No, your baby cannot catch cystitis in the sense that the bacteria travel to and infect the fetus. There is some evidence, however, that the tendency to have cystitis may be inherited.

CHAPTER 14

Children Get Cystitis, Too

We are in the midst of a scientific age when rapid gains are being made in determining hereditary basis for a great many diseases. We now know that children born to parents with cancer, heart disease, diabetes, allergies, and a host of other conditions are statistically more likely to have these same conditions. Still, the study of genetic predispositions remains pretty well centered on major diseases such as those mentioned. Few women worry—or even think about the fact—that their own predispositon to cystitis may show up in their daughters.

Certainly Fran never considered the possibility, even though she had dealt with recurring cystitis for a number of years before starting her own program of prevention, which reduced the number of episodes considerably. When Fran appeared in her pediatrician's office with her 5-year-old daughter, Lisa, one day, the pediatrician sensed right away that something was troubling the mother and daughter. "I wet my bed three times last week," Lisa announced without any fanfare. Fran picked up on the statement without missing a beat. "She was perfectly trained; hasn't wet her bed in more than three years. She started school a few weeks ago and she isn't especially fond of being in such a large group of children. She complains a lot when she comes home every day, and we have been trying to work out a way for her to accept the situation and try to make it better for herself. Now this has started. Do you think she is trying to let out her hostility over the school situation? Is she trying to punish me for something?"

The pediatrician began to question Lisa about her urinary habits: Did she have to urinate often (during the day at school? Did it hurt her in any way when she did urinate? Was she having any pain in her stomach? She asked Fran if Lisa's urine had a different look to it and if it had an odor that was unfamiliar and unpleasant? Did she ever notice blood in the child's urine? The series of "no's" to the questions gave some relief; there was probably not an infection going on. But what *was* causing Lisa's sudden reversal to the habit of bed-wetting, or enuresis, as it is medically termed?

The pediatrician's immediate concern about Lisa was that she might have had a bladder infection; such infections are not uncommon in childhood and they are 10 times more frequent in girls than in boys. About 5 percent of all girls will have one or more urinary tract infections before reaching maturity.

In most cases, except during infancy, it is not a physical abnormality that causes the onset of the infection, although this *is* the reason in about 5 percent of girls and 50 percent of boys with urinary tract infection. Most UTIs are caused by bacteria, just as is the case in adults. In Lisa's case, it was a matter of poor hygiene—not wiping herself properly after a bowel movement—that had already become habit. Other causes are inflammation of the vagina, foreign bodies in the bladder or urethra, and possibly severe constipation.

In the case of Lisa, the isolated incidence of bed-wetting might have been an important clue to bladder infection. Other symptoms include: urgency; frequency; pain on urination; dribbling of urine; daytime incontinence; foul-smelling, cloudy, or bloody urine; fever; abdominal or back pain; vomiting; and redness of the external genitalia. Sometimes there are no symptoms at all—a situation referred to as silent UTI. And if the infection goes untreated, the symptoms may disappear for a time, only to return later on.

How is bladder infection diagnosed in children? Much the same as in adults: with a urine culture. It is especially important that a child be monitored closely in giving a urine sample, becuase there is chance for contamination, which would confound the diagnosis. A search for obstruction in the urinary tract is undertaken only after two or three bouts of UTI or one bout with an infection that is resistant to treatment.

Should you institute home treatment with a young child? Let me repeat again that once an infection starts, there is no way to eradicate the infection except with antibiotic therapy. Children may respond and react to drugs much differently than do adults, and your doctor may ask you questions about your child's previous exprience with medications before settling upon a choice of therapy.

On the surface, it would seem that there is more of a potential for adverse or even toxic effects of medications in a child. Surprisingly, this is not always the case. In fact, as compared with adults, children seldom have serious adverse reactions to UTI antibiotics. There are several reasons why they are not more trouble free than adults: For one thing, drugs are usually prescribed on the basis of body weight, so large doses of a drug are seldom given. Second, there is usually not the danger of interference from other drugs or alcohol. Third, a child's kidney function is usually intact and therefore the drug is better metabolized than in some adults with compromised kidney funtion.

TEACH PREVENTION TO YOUR CHILD

How can you, a concerned parent (who may or may not suffer with cystitis) be sure that your child will enjoy a cystitis-free life? I can't think of a better time to launch a program of prevention of cystitis than in childhood when bad habits have not yet been acquired. Here are some suggestions:

- Teach your child—expecially your daughter—to wipe herself from the front to back after a bowel movement. Most children readily understand the difference between clean and not clean and the reasons for the practice should be spelled out carefully
- Teach your child to go to the bathroom whenever the urge to urinate starts. Children always want to finish the game, or the television program, or whatever. Answering the first signals to urinate should—and can—become second nature to a child, with your help. And set a good example.
- Teach your child to empty her bladder completely. A child will sometimes release the first spurt of urine, which will relieve the pressure, and then jump off the toilet to go on to something more exciting. Develop a few games, if necessary, to make the child give a final "push" to get the last drops of urine out.
- Teach your child to love cranberry juice. This is an acquired taste because of the slightly tart taste of cranberries. Some children love it immediately, and this is a plus. If there is resistance, try what one of my young mothers did: Fix a cranberry juice cocktail in a special glass with a cherry or some other decoration on top. This becomes a special treat for a child.

CHAPTER 15

Interstitial: The Other Cystitis

This is a relative newcomer to the list of disorders of the genitourinary tract, not because it is of recent origin, but because, in the past, doctors have tried to categorize it as some rare type of bacterial cystitis, which it is not.

Interstitial cystitis is an inflammation of the bladder wall. It is not a bacterial infection; in fact, the cause (and possible cures) are unknown. Women with interstitial cystitis have bladders that are chronically inflamed. Scar tissue forms all over the chronically inflamed bladder wall. Once the scar tissue forms, the bladder becomes stiff and inflexible and can no longer expand to its normal capacity. A bladder that once held 350 cubic centimeters of fluid (about the same size as a 12-ounce can of soda) is now reduced to as little as 50 cubic centimeters. The pressure of even the most minute amount of fluid becomes intolerable. Women with interstitial cystitis say that they sometimes have to urinate 60 or 70 times a day.

A key difference between interstitial and bacterial cystitis is in symptoms in urination itself. Whereas urine passing though the urethra may cause burning and pain for one with bacterial cystitis, it will bring a brief measure of relief to a person with interstitial cystitis. But the relief *is* brief, and often it is difficult for the victim of interstitial cystitis to feel that she has had any relief at all.

At one time, interstitial cystitis was thought to be a rare disease seen only in postmenopausal women. Today we are beginning to see cases in younger women, although the reasons for that are still as much a matter of speculation as the cause itself. It is estimated that some 500,000 adults suffer with interstitial cystitis in the United States alone, and 90 percent of these victims are women.

Theories abound about the origins of the disease; over the years, doctors have sought bacterial, drug reaction, and pyschiatric causes. At the moment, the consensus is that interstitial cystitis is an autoimmune disease in which the bladder lining is attacked by antibodies produced to battle some substance that the body perceives as foreign. Researchers believe that in women with interstitial cystitis, something in the urine sets off this autoimmune reaction. It is thought to be a genetic disease, which means that if you do have it, other women in your family have an increased risk of developing it as well.

Interstitial cystitis is difficult to diagnose. If urine cultures for bacteria come back from the laboratory negative, thus ruling out the usual causative organisms and other UTI mimickers such as chlamydia and mycoplasma are ruled out, I refer my patient to a urologist for additional tests. The urologist will first rule out possibilities such as multiple sclerosis and bladder cancer with a neurological examination of the bladder and other special tests. The true test, however, is a cystoscopy, a test that involves inserting a cystoscope (a specially lighted fiber-optic tube) through the urethra into the bladder. This is done under general anesthesia so there is no pain involved. As the bladder is filled with fluid, the cystoscopy will reveal the telltale signs: tiny red marks that represent pinpoint hemorrhages in the bladder wall. These are present even in the early stages of interstitial cystitis, before the bladder's capacity has been noticeably reduced.

I wish I could announce here that there is an easy cure

or reversal for interstitial cystitis, but such is not the case, at least not at the present time. What is available, however, are a number of treatments that sometimes provide remarkable relief for some women.

DMSO

This chemical—dimethylsulfoxide—is an industrial solvent that is also produced in medical grade. It has been approved by the Food and Drug Administration for use in interstitial cystitis. When instilled into the bladder, DMSO appears to act as an antiinflammatory agent and also dilates the blood vessels, providing pain relief in 70 to 80 percent of women who use it.

Chlorpactin

This Clorox-like drug also seems to work well for some women when instilled into the bladder. The theory is that it irritates the bladder lining to the extent that it destroys pain receptors, thus providing pain relief.

Silver Nitrate

This is another chemical that is instilled into the bladder and is believed to affect pain receptors. It should be understood, however, that this and the other treatments mentioned above only provide pain relief and do nothing to alter the course of the disease.

Bladder Distention

This method is also successful in some women although, because it is performed under general anesthesia, it is not done as a first-line treatment. In the procedure, the bladder (which is covered with scar tissue on the inside) is filled with air with a hydraulic device. This stretches the bladder, breaks up the existing scar tissue, and provides relief from pain.

Sodium Pentasanopolysulfate

This chemical is under study by researchers at present. When instilled into the bladder, it theoretically provides a protective lining to the inflamed bladder wall, thus preventing "acid burn," from urine.

Interstitial Cystitis Association

Perhaps the biggest leap in treating people with interstitial cystitis is the founding of self-help associations that offer sufferers contact with others who have the disease. One such group is the Interstitial Cystitis Association, co-founded by Dr. Vicki C. Ratner, an orthopedic resident at Montefiore Medical Center in New York City. Even as a part of the medical profession, Dr. Ratner was misdiagnosed for nearly two years before she finally had to research the symptoms on her own and then track down the few people who were doing research. When she insisted upon having a bladder distention and cystoscopy, the tiny hemorrhages became evident and her disease finally was confirmed.

The Interstitial Cystitis Association, with membership nationwide of nearly 10,000, provides members with much-needed support in the form of up-to-the-minute information via state coordinators and national quarterly newsletter. At present, its representatives are lobbying for funding by the National Institutes of Health in order to forge ahead with research into the causes of the debilitating disease.

Recently, the Association, in conjunction with the Urban Institute in Washington, D.C., conducted a pilot study of interstitial cystitis sufferers. The emerging portrait is one of a devastating disease. Of those surveyed, 40 percent had lost their jobs because of their illness, 27 percent had lost spouses or lovers, 55 percent had considered suicide, 12 percent had actually attempted it, and 45 percent had to see five or more doctors before they were properly diagnosed.

The Association, however, does not promise a cure at this date. As Dr. Ratner has put it, "That would be a false hope." What is available is the support of other interstitial cystitis sufferers who often come together in groups to disseminate information and share experiences. This kind of relating, I think, is invaluable because it gives the victim of *any* disease a sense of control. As I have stressed throughout this book, control is a major part of the battle over a medical condition that threatens to disrupt your life.

It is my optimistic hope that the cause of interstitial cystitis will soon be discovered and that this discovery will be quickly followed by a cure or cures, and even a program of prevention. For now, it is my hope that victims of interstitial cystitis will seek the help that *is* available: from doctors who can offer very effective symptomatic pain relief and from the Interstitial Cystitis Association, which can offer resources and information.

For further information write to The Interstitial Cystitis Association, P.O. Box 1553, Madison Square Station, New York, NY 10159.

Epilogue

Recently, in my files, I came across a newspaper clipping from a few years back. The clipping is frayed at the edges and slightly yellow, but I keep it because it is a happy reminder of how my cystitis prevention program got its start. The clipping listed the medical reasons why people stay home from work. It said that, according to a survey, cystitis is one of the most common causes of absenteeism among women, second only to the upper respiratory infection. A short note attached to the clipping was signed by Mona S. It read, simply: "I'll bet this is no news to you."

Based on my own recollections of women whose jobs had been seriously affected by cystitis, I was not at all surprised by the report in the newspaper. At the time, in fact, I felt that it stopped short of making a very important observation. Cystitis not only causes women to be physically absent from their work, but in a larger sense it also causes them to miss out on life. The physical symptoms of cystitis—the constant urge to urinate, burning, and pain—are impossible to ignore.

For the lucky woman, an attack of cystitis means a few days on medication, then the problem is over, never to return again. But for the vast majority of women who have it, cystitis is a source of constant irritation and frustration. Mona was counted among the latter group. Her cystitis attacks, which began when she was about 22 years old, were severe and debilitating and did, indeed, cause her to take valuable time away from her work. But as bothersome as the attacks were, equally as troublesome were the days spent in anticipation of an attack, days planned and lived with cystitis as her frame of reference.

Mona's first visit to me for treatment coincided with those of a number of other women who had endured one cystitis attack after another. Listening to them recount their experiences with treatment and the inevitable return of the disease started me thinking that the only certain "cure" for cystitis is to stop it before it starts—with a program of prevention.

I decided to enhance the traditional treatment of that small group of women with the prevention program that has evolved into this book. It was certainly not a difficult regimen. Most of the components, as we have seen, involve simple lifestyle changes. The women welcomed the opportunity to go a step beyond conventional drug treatment, which for them had not been successful on a long-term basis. Now, three years later, I am happy to say that Mona and the other women in that pioneer program come to my office only for their regular gynecological checkups, not for what once seemed to be never-ending cystitis attacks.

Of all the many women who have found relief from their chronic cystitis, Mona remains the most enthusiastic proponent of the preventive measures that have kept her cystitis-free for more than three years. While we worked together to create an individualized set of lifestyle changes for her, Mona began to develop a new perspective on her disease. She came to realize that the cystitis had become magnified out of proportion to other aspects of her life, and was able, eventually to regain control.

Perhaps, like Mona, you have felt overpowered by this disease, at a loss over what to do next. What you have found in these pages is a plan that will put you in control of the condition, a plan that could, as it did for Mona and thousands of other women, help you win your battle with cystitis forever.

Index